# Asthma Management

## Clinical Pathways, Guidelines, and Patient Education

### Health & Administration Development Group

**Jo Gulledge**
Executive Director

**Shawn Beard**
Research Editor

**AN ASPEN PUBLICATION®**
Aspen Publishers, Inc.
Gaithersburg, Maryland
1999

ASPEN CHRONIC DISEASE MANAGEMENT SERIES

Library of Congress Cataloging-in-Publication Data

Asthma management : clinical pathways, guidelines, and patient
education / Health & Administration Development Group;
Jo Gulledge, executive director; Shawn Beard, research editor.
p. cm. — (Aspen chronic disease management series)
Includes index.
ISBN: 0-8342-1705-8
1. Asthma Handbooks, manuals, etc. 2. Medical protocols
Handbooks, manuals, etc. 3. Patient education Handbooks,
manuals, etc. I. Gulledge, Jo. II. Beard, Shawn. III. Health and
Administration Development Group (Aspen Publishers) IV. Series.
[DNLM: 1. Asthma—therapy. 2. Asthma—diagnosis.
3. Critical Pathways. 4. Patient Education.
WF 553 A85475 1999]
RC591.A825 1999
616.2'38—dc21
DNLM/DLC
for Library of Congress
99-31841 CIP

Editorial Services: Marsha Davies

Copyright © 1999 by Aspen Publishers, Inc.

Orders: (800) 638-8437
Customer Service: (800) 234-1660

**About Aspen Publishers** • For more than 35 years, Aspen has been a leading professional
publisher in a variety of disciplines. Aspen's vast information resources are available in both
print and electronic formats. We are committed to providing the highest quality information
available in the most appropriate format for our customers. Visit Aspen's Internet site for more
information resources, directories, articles, and a searchable version of Aspen's full catalog,
including the most recent publications: **http://www.aspenpublishers.com**
**Aspen Publishers, Inc.** • The hallmark of quality in publishing
Member of the worldwide Wolters Kluwer group

Library of Congress Catalog Card Number: 99-31841
ISBN: 0-8342-1705-8

Printed in the United States of America

1 2 3 4 5

# Table of Contents

# Editorial Board

**Claire B. Rossé, RN, BS, MBA**
Founder and CEO
FutureHealth Corporation
Timonium, Maryland

**Rachel Stipe, RN, BS, CPHQ**
Quality Improvement/Reimbursement Specialist
Spectracare, Inc.
Louisville, Kentucky

**Maura J. Sughrue, MD**
Medical Director
Fairfax Family Practice Centers
Fairfax, Virginia

**Warren E. Todd, MBA**
Vice President, Business Development
Hastings Healthcare Group
Pennington, New Jersey

**Marcus D. Wilson, PharmD**
President
Health Core, Inc.
Newark, Delaware

# Introduction

Disease management is based on the understanding that a small proportion of the population—individuals with chronic conditions—consumes the vast majority of health care resources. Focusing on chronic illnesses, disease management programs strive to reduce costly hospitalizations through continual, rather than episodic, care. The logic is straightforward: providing a continuum of care dramatically reduces the incidence of acute episodes requiring inpatient treatment.

Because of disease management's emphasis on continual care, effective education of patients, families, and other informal caregivers is a vital component. Providers form partnerships with patients and families, teaching them to take daily responsibility for managing disease.

Asthma is one of several chronic disease states affecting millions of Americans. In fact, asthma is the most common chronic condition of children. Because of its prevalence and gravity, it is imperative to create a disease-management program that aids clinicians in diagnosing and effectively controlling the disease.

*Asthma Management* provides comprehensive, detailed guidelines on all aspects of managing asthma from the initial diagnosis in the clinical examination to the treatment strategy, which may include drug therapy and lifestyle modification. *Asthma Management* couples these clinical guidelines with patient education handouts, which teach patients to comply with interventions, while also learning the principles of demand management: recognizing and prioritizing their health care needs. Through education, patients know when professional interventions are required and use resources accordingly.

To ensure quick access to the information clinicians need most, *Asthma Management* is divided into two parts.

Part I, "Managing Asthma: Clinical Pathways and Guidelines," addresses the essentials of administering asthma management programs, with information on developing and implementing clinical guidelines/pathways, measuring and managing outcomes, and monitoring and improving patient satisfaction. While the guidelines originate from nationally recognized sources, their purpose is to serve as a starting point for providers and payers pursuing disease management. They are meant to be adapted to meet the needs of specific populations and to be further refined for individual patients.

Part II, "Self-Management of Asthma: Patient Education," recognizes the patient education component of disease management. Consisting entirely of large-print patient handouts, including Spanish-language patient information sheets, this section is designed for clinicians across the care continuum to distribute freely to patients. The educational materials encourage patients and their families to become active partners in managing chronic conditions.

*Asthma Management* is not intended to add new information to the abundant literature relevant to disease management, but rather to extract from hundreds of publications the most sound and useful information available. The goal is to provide this information in such a manner that is concise, practical, and pertinent. To that end, *Asthma Management* distills the traditional narrative text and presents it in a quick-read format.

*Shawn K. Beard*
Research Editor
Health & Administration Development Group

# Acknowledgments

Creating a reference volume such as *Asthma Management* demands tremendous effort during the development period—shaping the manual's focus, collecting and evaluating materials, and ensuring that the format is practical and easy to use.

Foremost among the people who help us fulfill these responsibilities are the editorial board members. By answering queries, providing contacts, and reviewing materials, they play an instrumental role in the development of a high quality resource.

I am grateful to all the health care facilities, organizations, individual professionals, and others who generously shared their clinical guidelines, pathways, and patient education materials with us—special thanks to Pediatric Services of America, Norcross, Georgia; Thomas F. Plaut, MD, Amherst, Massachusetts; and American Academy of Allergy, Asthma and Immunology, Milwaukee, Wisconsin.

In addition, this project never could have progressed from a bare-bones idea to a comprehensive resource without the untiring support of Rosemarie Cooper, Administrative Assistant; the skill of Marsha Davies, Editorial Services, and the guidance of Jo Gulledge, Executive Director, Health & Administration Development Group.

*Shawn Beard*
Research Editor
Health & Administration Development Group

# Tracking Form

**POLICY**

Patient education documentation

**PURPOSE**

To provide interdisciplinary documentation of patient/family education

**PROCEDURE**

1. On admission, stamp the Tracking Form with patient's Addressograph plate and place in front of chart.
2. Within first three days of admission, have licensed nursing/therapy staff identify patient/family educational needs.
3. Read and follow directions 1–3 on the Tracking Form.
4. Fill out specific sections of the Tracking Form.

- **Document:** List of materials from manual by chapter.
- **Initial/Date Given:** As material is given, initial and date in the space provided.
- **Primary Caregiver:** Indicate who is receiving education information (the caregiver or the patient).
- **Comments:** Write comments regarding when material was reviewed (provide date/initials), with whom, and any required special needs.
- **Demonstrates Understanding of Activity:** Initial and date when primary caregiver has demonstrated understanding of activity (must be completed before discharge).
- **Other Classes Attended:** List other education opportunities (classes attended and additional handouts) not already listed

5. Sign full name, with initials and title, on back of form.

Place Facility Logo Here

**Asthma Management**

DIRECTIONS:

1. Highlight APPROPRIATE patient education materials.
2. Initial and date when material was given/reviewed/completed.
3. Use comments column for:
   a. Charting dates reviewed.
   b. Special patient/family needs.
   c. Receiver of education.

ADDRESSOGRAPH

| DOCUMENT | Init/Date Given | Primary Caregiver | COMMENTS<br>Init/Dates Material Reviewed • Special Needs • Who Received Education | Init/Date States &/or Demonstrates Understanding of Activity | |
|---|---|---|---|---|---|
| **4. Overview of Asthma and Its Symptoms** | | | | | |
| About Asthma | | | | | |
| What Is Asthma? | | | | | |
| Common Questions and Answers about Asthma | | | | | |
| Datos sobre el asma | | | | | |
| Controlling Your Asthma | | | | | |
| Is Your Asthma under Control? | | | | | |
| ¿Está su asma bajo control? | | | | | |
| Cómo controlar las cosas que empeoran su asma | | | | | |
| About Peak Flow Meters | | | | | |
| How To Use Your Peak Flow Meter | | | | | |
| El medidor de flujo espiratorio máximo—Un termómetro para el asma | | | | | |
| Peak Flow Chart | | | | | |
| My Asthma Symptoms and Peak Flow Diary | | | | | |
| How To Stop Asthma Attacks from Happening | | | | | |
| How To Stay Away from Things That Make Your Asthma Worse | | | | | |
| Removing House Dust and Other Allergic Irritants from Your Home | | | | | |
| Desencadenantes de asma | | | | | |
| Patient Self-Assessment Form for Environmental and Other Factors That Can Make Asthma Worse | | | | | |
| Talking to People about Asthma | | | | | |

| DOCUMENT | Init/Date Given | Primary Caregiver | COMMENTS<br>Init/Dates Material Reviewed • Special Needs • Who Received Education | Init/Date States &/or Demonstrates Understanding of Activity |
|---|---|---|---|---|
| Check Your Asthma IQ | | | | |
| Worksheet: What To Expect from Your Asthma Treatment—The Goals | | | | |
| Patient Self-Assessment Form for Follow-Up Visits | | | | |
| **5. Medications for Asthma** | | | | |
| Medicines for Asthma | | | | |
| Asthma Medicines for (Name of Patient) | | | | |
| My Asthma Medicines | | | | |
| Beta$_2$-agonists | | | | |
| Theophylline | | | | |
| Cromolyn | | | | |
| Corticosteroids | | | | |
| How To Use a Spray Inhaler | | | | |
| Your Metered-Dose Inhaler—How To Use It | | | | |
| Medicamentos inhalados para el asma | | | | |
| Spacers—Making Inhaled Medicines Easier To Take | | | | |
| How To Use and Care for Your Nebulizer | | | | |
| **6. Managing Asthma Attacks** | | | | |
| Warning Signs of Asthma Episodes | | | | |
| What To Do for an Asthma Attack | | | | |
| Summary of Steps To Manage Asthma Episodes | | | | |
| Sample Patient Asthma Management Plan | | | | |
| Write a Plan for Controlling Your Asthma | | | | |
| Pocket-Size Asthma Action Plan | | | | |
| **7. Asthma and Staying Active** | | | | |
| Plan for Staying Active—for Children | | | | |
| How To Set Guidelines for Your Child's Activities | | | | |
| Plan for Staying Active—for Adults | | | | |
| Clues for Deciding To Go to School or Work | | | | |
| Helping Students Control Their Asthma | | | | |

| DOCUMENT | Init/Date Given | Primary Caregiver | COMMENTS Init/Dates Material Reviewed • Special Needs • Who Received Education | | Init/Date States &/or Demonstrates Understanding of Activity |
|---|---|---|---|---|---|
| **8. Asthma in Special Populations** | | | | | |
| If You Have Asthma and You Are Pregnant | | | | | |
| If You Have Asthma and You Are Over Age 55 | | | | | |
| If Your Infant Has Asthma, You Will Have To Take Extra Care | | | | | |
| Occupational Asthma | | | | | |
| Asma ocupacional | | | | | |
| Exercise-Induced Asthma and Bronchospasm | | | | | |
| Asma inducida por ejercicio y broncoespasmo | | | | | |
| **9. Patient Pathway and Care Planning Forms** | | | | | |
| Patient Pathway for Pediatric Ambulatory Asthma— 4/5 Years and Older | | | | | |
| Sample Care Path: Patient Version | | | | | |
| Sample Patient Standard of Care Information Sheet | | | | | |

| OTHER CLASSES ATTENDED/HANDOUTS GIVEN | INIT | SIGNATURE |
|---|---|---|
| | | |
| | | |
| | | |
| | | |
| | | |

# PART I

# Managing Asthma: Clinical Pathways and Guidelines

# 1. Asthma and Disease Management

## CHILDHOOD ASTHMA AND DISEASE MANAGEMENT*

### Importance

Asthma is the most common childhood chronic condition with an estimated prevalence rate between 5% and 10%. Asthma accounts for 23% of school absence days and remains one of the primary reasons for hospitalizing children. Children with severe asthma miss more than twice as many school days as healthy children. Data from the National Health Interview Survey suggest that the prevalence of asthma in the pediatric population increased by 29% between 1980 and 1987. Moreover, the hospitalization rates for children less than 15 years of age with asthma have increased substantially over the past 20 years. Of even greater concern is the 46% increase in death rates from asthma that were reported between 1980 and 1989 despite therapeutic advances in diagnosis and treatment.

### Efficacy or Effectiveness of Interventions

Research and clinical data indicate that effective treatment exists for children with asthma. The goals of asthma management are to: (1) maximize functional status of children as indicated by their ability to participate in normal activities; (2) maximize symptom relief (ie, minimize frequency of attacks, maximize pulmonary function); (3) facilitate child and family empowerment by maximizing self-efficacy in symptom control and treatment regimens; and (4) limit side effects of treatments and interventions.

### NHLBI and AAP Guidelines

The National Heart, Lung, and Blood Institute (NHLBI) issued guidelines for the diagnosis and management of asthma, including childhood asthma, in 1991. Guidelines were established for different clinical presentations of asthma and for different health care settings. Subsequently, an American Academy of Pediatrics (AAP) quality committee developed a practice parameter for the office-based management of acute exacerbations of childhood asthma. Critics of the 1991

guidelines have emphasized the lack of scientific rigor in their development and challenges in complying with the required structural elements; nonetheless, these guidelines became the national standard for asthma care.

The NHLBI revised its guidelines in 1997. Highlights of the 1997 guidelines appear in this chapter.

### Potential for Improving Quality

There are no national estimates about the extent to which current practice is consistent with the practice guidelines available from the NHLBI and the AAP. However, increases in the death rate over a time when therapeutic interventions were improving suggest that there is a potential for improving care. Studies of practice patterns in teaching hospitals and emergency rooms suggest that there is considerable variability in the management of acute exacerbations. A trial of an educational intervention in Los Angeles had to be discontinued because of the poor treatment being provided to children enrolled in the study. Some studies of medication regimens and self-management programs have shown reductions of greater than 50% in attack rates, emergency room use, and lost school days.

### Cost-Effectiveness of Interventions

No formal cost-effectiveness analyses were found. Certainly, improved management of asthma in the outpatient setting that contributes to reductions in emergency room and hospital use will be more cost-effective than strategies that lead to uncontrollable exacerbations. There are likely to be cost differences among the different medical therapies, but there is not much variation in the recommended strategies, suggesting that cost-effectiveness may not be much of a consideration in chronic management.

### Health Plan Role in Providing Intervention

The health plan has a role in the assessment and treatment of children with asthma. Perhaps as important, however, teaching parents and children how to manage this disease is likely to make a substantial contribution to improved outcomes. When a significant patient role is required, there is often a debate about the appropriate level of attribution to the health plan. Because parents and children cannot be expected to learn about self-management on their own, testing knowledge, attitudes, and beliefs of families and children with asthma may provide an indicator of the success of the health plan in communicating the necessary information.

*Source: Elizabeth A. McGlynn, "Choosing Chronic Disease Measures for HEDIS: Conceptual Framework and Review of Seven Clinical Areas," *Managed Care Quarterly*, Vol. 4:3, Aspen Publishers, Inc., © 1996.

## Areas for Quality Measurement Development

1. Appropriateness of medications prescribed for chronic management of asthma
2. Proportion of children and families with asthma who have adequate knowledge about the disease, control of symptoms, elimination of environmental triggers, and a plan for dealing with an acute exacerbation
3. Adequacy of office resources for management of an acute exacerbation
4. Appropriateness of hospitalization and emergency room visits for asthma

## ADOLESCENT REFRACTORY ASTHMA AND DISEASE MANAGEMENT*

Less than 5% of asthmatics are classified as severe, and nearly half the claims costs for all asthmatics occur in the emergency department and hospital. More important is the observation that only 10% to 20% of asthmatics receive inhaled steroids, considered the cornerstone of therapy. The reason appears to be that inhaled bronchodilators are overused because of their ability to provide instant relief. Finally, physicians are not the most frequently encountered caregiver. Asthmatics see their pharmacists five times more often. This has raised the position of the pharmacist in disease management programs to that of a true provider and educator, sometimes with financial incentives. Ironically, this opportunity is lost when subscribers are financially motivated to use mail order programs for inhaler refills. Compensatory efforts include visits by home nurses specializing in asthma and various phone and mail prompts.

The entire continuum of asthma care is displayed in the exhibit, "Continuum of Care for Adolescent Refractory Asthma." The contrast between a hospital-based case manager's role and that of the disease manager is dramatic.

## Results

Results from individual delivery system implementation of disease management for asthma are consistent over all regions in the United States. The most important observations include the following:

- reduction in hospitalizations by half or more
- reduction in emergency department visits by half or more
- abrupt increase in the use of inhaled steroids
- decrease in reliance on bronchodilators
- improved functional status, as measured by:
  - ability to work
  - quality of sleep

---

*Source: David W. Plocher, "Disease Management," in Peter R. Kongstvedt, ed., *The Managed Health Care Handbook*, 3d ed., Aspen Publishers, Inc., © 1996.

## CONTINUUM OF CARE FOR ADOLESCENT REFRACTORY ASTHMA

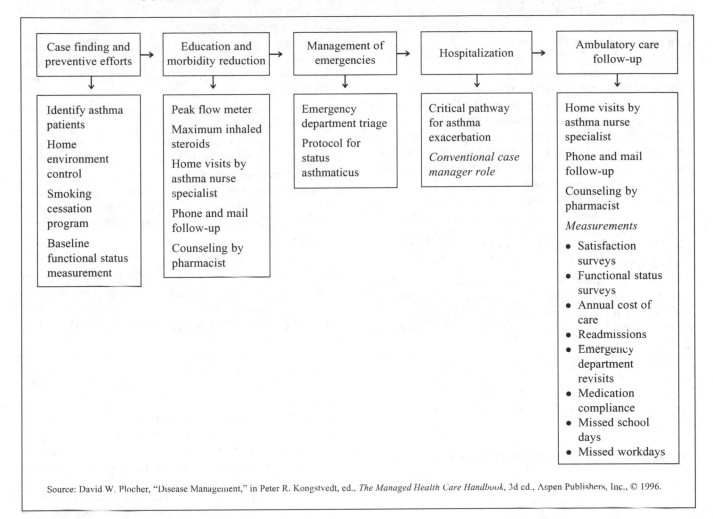

Source: David W. Plocher, "Disease Management," in Peter R. Kongstvedt, ed., *The Managed Health Care Handbook*, 3d ed., Aspen Publishers, Inc., © 1996.

## CLINICIAN EDUCATION—MYTHS AND FACTS ABOUT ASTHMA MANAGEMENT*

### Early Diagnosis of Asthma

**Belief:** The diagnosis of asthma will frighten and upset patients.

**Fact:** Absence of the diagnosis will deprive parents or patients of the opportunity to learn about asthma and intervene early in the course of an attack.

**Solution:** Describe asthma as an illness with a broad range of severity. Parents will be reassured to hear that most cases are mild.

### Early Use of Oral Steroids

**Belief:** Overuse may cause serious side effects.

**Fact:** Oral steroids are the most potent medicine available to treat inflammation during an attack. Concern with overuse leads to underuse: thus many patients who would benefit from oral steroids do not get them. As a result, they will require emergency care or admission to the hospital where they will receive high doses of steroids.

**Solution:** Describe the 1988 study that shows early use of steroids decreased hospitalizations by 90% in an experi-

*Source: Thomas F. Plaut, "A Systems Approach to Asthma Care," *Managed Care Quarterly*, Vol. 4:3, Aspen Publishers, Inc., © 1996.

mental group. Because these patients had fewer serious episodes, they used less steroids than the control group.

## Use of Inhalation Devices

Compressor-driven nebulizer:

**Belief:** Home administration of an adrenaline-like medicine by compressor-driven nebulizer is dangerous because a parent might treat too often and cause toxicity.

**Fact:** The major danger of using the compressor-driven nebulizer at home is that it can mask symptoms. An inadequately instructed patient or parent will not recognize that the asthma is going out of control.

**Solution:** Give patients a home treatment plan based on the asthma care zones as determined by peak flow or asthma signs. This will limit the frequency of use and will direct parents at what point to see the doctor.

Holding chamber:

**Belief:** Most patients who use metered-dose inhalers (MDIs) will not benefit from using a holding chamber.

**Fact:** The holding chamber increases the benefits of inhaled steroids and decreases the side effects of all medicines delivered by MDI.

**Solution:** Ask physician to demonstrate proper MDI use with and without holding chamber during hands-on practice. The physician will appreciate the difficulty patients have in using the MDI alone and the ease of its use with a holding chamber.

## Objective Monitoring of Patient Status

Monitoring peak flow:

**Belief:** An asthma symptom diary is just as good as a peak flow diary in helping patients manage asthma.

**Fact:** Peak flow often drops before symptoms occur. The peak flow meter is the best tool for assessing asthma at home.

**Solution:** The Asthma Peak Flow Diary, which includes both peak flow scores and symptoms, can serve as an educational, monitoring, and management tool for patients over four years of age.

Monitoring asthma signs:

**Belief:** Parents are not competent to assess asthma symptoms in children under five.

**Fact:** Well-trained parents can accurately assess their child's status.

**Solution:** Provide asthma assessment system based on signs that parents can hear and see, using the Asthma Signs Diary.

## Daily Preventive Treatment

**Belief:** Only about 10% of asthma patients need to take preventive medicine daily.

**Fact:** About 40% of asthma patients, practically all those with symptoms more than two days per week, will benefit from daily preventive medicine.

**Solution:** Encourage physicians to prescribe preventive treatment for their patients with moderate asthma while tracking them with an asthma diary. They will be impressed with the results.

## Education

**Belief:** Prescribing medicines is much more important than providing asthma education.

**Fact:** Many asthma patients take their medicines improperly and derive little benefit from them. Patients who do not understand what triggers their asthma attacks cannot prevent them.

**Solution:** Teach doctors the correct techniques for taking medicines and ways that patients can avoid their asthma triggers.

## MANAGEMENT OF ACUTE ASTHMA IN CHILDREN*

### Pathogenesis

Reversible airway obstruction is the hallmark of asthma. Contributing to the obstruction are bronchiolar smooth muscle contraction, inflammation, and edema. The asthmatic airway exhibits an exaggerated response to a variety of stimuli, including allergens, infections, and exercise. This hyperresponsiveness is generated by the release of chemical mediators (histamines, prostaglandins, and leukotrienes) from inflammatory cells (mast cells, eosinophils, lymphocytes, and macrophages).

### Clinical Evaluation

In the assessment of the child with acute wheezing, the treating physician should first obtain a brief, focused history followed by examination of the chest and administration of treatment. The initial history should include questions regarding the onset of wheezing (i.e., abrupt or subacute), its duration, the severity of distress compared with previous attacks, and medications recently taken.

Once treatment has begun, a more comprehensive history may be obtained. The names, doses, and frequency of asthma medications recently received should be identified. The

*Source: Tom Stein, MD, FACEP, and Richard Scarfone, MD, "Management of Acute Asthma in Children," *Topics in Emergency Medicine*, Vol. 18:3, Aspen Publishers, Inc., © September 1996.

presence or absence of fever should be noted. A history of difficulty sleeping, eating, or speaking as a result of this attack suggests a severe exacerbation. In addition, questions regarding the hydration status of the child (fluid intake and urine output) should be asked. If this patient is wheezing for the first time, then inquiries regarding other possible causes of wheezing (see below) should be made. For those with previous bouts of wheezing, prior hospitalizations or admissions to the intensive care unit would be notable. Family history should focus on asthma, cystic fibrosis, or atopic disease.

## Physical Examination

The physical assessment of the wheezing child should initially focus on level of consciousness, vital signs, and pulmonary examination. A child who is anxious, restless, or lethargic may be hypoxemic. The heart rate, respiratory rate, and oxygen saturation should be noted. The child's degree of wheezing should be ascertained by auscultation. In children with severe disease, wheezing may be audible without a stethoscope; if aeration is extremely poor, no wheezing may be detected. In addition, the inspiratory-to-expiratory ratio should be recorded; a prolonged expiratory phase indicates extreme bronchospasm. The child's use of accessory muscles will indicate the work of breathing. Asymmetric wheezing suggests pneumonia, pneumothorax, or the presence of a foreign body. Palpation of the chest and neck may reveal subcutaneous air associated with a pneumomediastinum.

After this initial assessment, the remainder of the physical examination may be performed. It is prudent to delay performing the most anxiety-provoking aspects of the examination (e.g., otoscopy) until after treatment has begun.

## Differential Diagnosis

Although most children with wheezing have asthma, other conditions must be considered. Bronchiolitis is a disease of the lower respiratory tract seen predominantly in the winter and frequently manifesting as wheezing in infants and young toddlers. Viruses, particularly respiratory syncytial virus, are the most common cause. Typically there is a 2- to 3-day prodrome of low-grade fever, rhinorrhea, or cough followed by tachypnea, retractions, and wheezing. Thus asthma and bronchiolitis usually cannot be distinguished on physical examination findings alone. An infant who has never wheezed before, however, or one who presents with an upper respiratory tract infection and wheezing in the winter probably has bronchiolitis. Many of these patients will respond to ß₂-agonists; corticosteroids have not been shown to be efficacious, however, and their routine use in bronchiolitis should be discouraged.

Foreign body aspiration is most common in children aged 1 to 5 years. Although the onset of symptomatology may be insidious, this diagnosis should be strongly suspected in a toddler with no history of asthma who has localized wheezing after an episode of choking. Diagnosis may be aided by inspiratory/expiratory or lateral decubitus radiographs, fluoroscopy, or rigid bronchoscopy.

Gastroesophageal reflux presents most commonly in early infancy. For a small subset of children, poor lower esophageal sphincter function results in regurgitation and aspiration of gastric contents, leading to reflex bronchospasm. The diagnosis should be suspected in the young infant with recurrent wheezing, especially if there is a history of frequent "spitting up" or failure to thrive.

The diagnosis of cystic fibrosis is established during infancy in about 50% of affected children. This autosomal recessive condition is found most commonly, but not exclusively, in white children. Although the degree of illness is extremely variable, many patients will have recurrent exacerbations of coughing, wheezing, and respiratory distress. Other clues to the diagnosis are recurrent pneumonia, large malodorous stools, a salty taste to the skin, and failure to thrive.

After exposure to an antigen, children with anaphylaxis may have an abrupt onset of wheezing and stridor, often associated with a urticarial rash and hypotension. Recent medication use or exposure to certain foods (eggs, nuts, or shellfish) or bee venom suggests the diagnosis.

## Laboratory Studies

Pulse oximetry is a noninvasive means to obtain objective data regarding the degree of illness of a wheezing child. The initial arterial oxygen saturation ($SaO_2$), as measured by pulse oximetry, has been shown to predict the need for hospitalization among children in the emergency department (ED) with acute asthma. Furthermore, in another study there was a poor correlation between the physician's clinical assessment of the degree of illness and that reflected by the $SaO_2$. Thus the $SaO_2$ should be determined for all moderately or severely ill children soon after ED arrival as an adjunct to the physical examination. Supplemental oxygen should be provided for those with a level of 95% or less. A delay of at least 10 minutes after a ß₂-agonist treatment delivered in 100% oxygen is necessary to obtain an accurate $SaO_2$ in room air. Asthmatics are not at risk for developing hypercarbia from oxygen therapy.

With the advent of pulse oximetry, it is usually unnecessary to measure arterial blood gases solely to determine the partial pressure of oxygen. If there is concern about impending respiratory failure, then a measurement of the partial pressure of carbon dioxide ($Paco_2$) can be helpful. One must be careful to interpret such data in light of the clinical picture. For example, a "normal" $Paco_2$ of 40 mm Hg in a child with a respiratory rate of 66 breath/min and significant retractions suggests impaired ventilation and impending respiratory failure.

For older children, it is helpful to measure the peak expiratory flow. This provides objective data regarding the degree of respiratory compromise and, along with other clinical parameters, can be used to assess the child's response to therapy. For young children, however, the usefulness of this measurement is somewhat limited because they often cannot reliably perform this effort-dependent maneuver.

The decision to obtain a chest radiograph should be made on the basis of clinical findings. Hyperinflation, interstitial infiltrates, and streaky atelectasis are common radiographic findings in patients who are wheezing. Less commonly, a serious condition associated with asthma, such as pneumonia, pneumomediastinum, or pneumothorax, may be seen. Rarely is an unsuspected diagnosis made on the basis of a chest radiograph in the acutely wheezing child. In one study of children who were wheezing for the first time, 95% of chest radiographs obtained were normal. Among those children with abnormal films, 95% would have been identified had radiographs been limited to those with focal chest findings, fever, or extreme tachypnea or tachycardia. Thus it should not be a routine practice to obtain a chest film for all wheezing children.

## Treatment

### $ß_2$-Agonists

All patients with an acute asthma attack should receive a $ß_2$-agonist on entry into the emergency medical system (see "Medications for the Treatment of Acute Asthma." Albuterol, a selective $ß_2$-agonist with a relatively long half-life, is the drug of choice. The preferred route of administration is by inhalation; peak effect is within minutes, and adverse effects are minimal. Although handheld nebulizers are most commonly employed, delivery of $ß_2$-agonists by metered-dose inhalers with a spacing device has been shown to be at least as effective and is more cost effective when treating mild to moderate attacks. A face mask–equipped spacer may be effectively employed for children too young to use the metered-dose inhaler properly. When a nebulizer is used, it is preferable to employ a mouthpiece rather than a face mask to avoid nasal deposition of the drug.

For severely ill children, options include delivering $ß_2$-agonists either parenterally or by continuous nebulization or by administering sympathomimetics subcutaneously. Continuously nebulized drug delivery has been studied primarily in children and has been found to be safe and possibly more effective than intermittent drug administration. Muscle cramping, hypokalemia, and hyperglycemia are possible complications but are usually not clinically important. Extremely dyspneic children with a poor peak flow who show a suboptimal response to initial $ß_2$-agonist nebulizations may need to receive epinephrine or terbutaline subcutaneously or $ß_2$-agonists intravenously in an attempt to achieve bronchodilation. These patients must be observed closely for tachycardia, dysrhythmias, and hypertension.

### Corticosteroids

For many years, it was believed that the onset of clinical effects from corticosteroids was too delayed for them to be clinically useful in the acute treatment of status asthmaticus. There are now compelling data, however, showing that their prompt use can decrease the need for hospitalization. In one study, oral prednisone was shown to reduce the need for hospitalization among children treated aggressively with $ß_2$-agonists; this benefit was achieved within 4 hours of prednisone administration. Oral prednisone has other advantages in that it is rapidly and completely absorbed, can be given before hospital admission if necessary, and causes fewer of the minor complications often associated with parenteral therapy. Most important, routine use of prednisone for all moderately ill children in the ED will avoid delays in corticosteroid delivery in the ED pending the insertion of an intravenous line.

It follows, then, that oral administration would result in an increased utilization of corticosteroids in the ED, especially among children. Inhaled dexamethasone also has been shown to be effective in this patient population. If discharged, however, these patients may need to be continued on oral steroid therapy. Likewise, intravenous steroids may be given, but they are probably not cost effective if one follows these guidelines.

The National Institutes of Health Expert Panel report (see Chapter 2) recommends that corticosteroids be given to any asthmatic child who does not improve after 1 hour of $ß_2$-agonist therapy. Given that clinical benefits from steroids are delayed and that all moderately ill children will require steroids whether or not they require hospitalization, however, it seems more prudent to administer steroids soon after ED arrival in an attempt to hasten clinical improvement and perhaps prevent the need for hospitalization.

### Aminophylline

Aminophylline has been relegated to adjunctive therapy for acute and chronic asthma management. Aminophylline increases the toxicity but not the efficacy of inhaled $ß_2$-agonists.

## MEDICATIONS FOR THE TREATMENT OF ACUTE ASTHMA

| Drug | Route | Recommended dose or dosage | Maximum dose or dosage | Dosing instructions |
|------|-------|---------------------------|------------------------|---------------------|
| Albuterol (intermittent) | Nebulization | 0.15 mg/kg | 5.0 mg | Repeat every 20–30 minutes |
| Albuterol (continuous) | Nebulization | 0.5 mg/kg/hour | 15 mg/hour | |
| Epinephrine (1 mg/mL) | Subcutaneous | 0.01 mL/kg/hour | 0.3 mL (1:1000) | May be repeated every 15–20 minutes |
| Ipratropium bromide | Nebulization | 250 µg | | |
| Magnesium sulfate | Intravenous | 40–50 mg/kg | | Over 20 minutes |
| Methylprednisolone | Intravenous/oral | 2 mg/kg | 125 mg | |
| Prednisone | Oral | 2 mg/kg | 60 mg | |
| Terbutaline (1 mg/mL) | Subcutaneous | 0.01 mL/kg/hour | 0.3 mL (1:1000) | May be repeated every 15–20 minutes |
| Terbutaline | Bolus | 10 µg/kg over 10 minutes, then 0.4 µg/kg/min infusion | 0.4 µg/kg/min infusion | May rebolus every 30 minutes with 10 µg/kg and increase infusion by 0.2 µg/kg/min |
| Glycopyrrolate | Nebulization | 1 mg every 6 hours | | |
| Dexamethasone | Nebulization | 1.5 mg/kg | | |

Source: Tom Stein, MD, FACEP, and Richard Scarfone, MD, "Management of Acute Asthma in Children," *Topics in Emergency Medicine,* Vol. 18:3, Aspen Publishers, Inc., © September 1996.

### Anticholinergics

Stimulation of airway cholinergic receptors results in reflex bronchoconstriction and may be blocked with the use of anticholinergic agents such as atropine. The use of anticholinergics has increased since the advent of ipratropium bromide, which because it is poorly absorbed has fewer systemic anticholinergic effects than atropine. Anticholinergic agents have a slower onset of action compared with ß$_2$-agonists, but their action is more prolonged. Ipratropium is available as a metered-dose inhaler as well as a solution for nebulization. Some studies have shown that the use of ß$_2$-agonists with ipratroprium is more effective than the use of ß$_2$-agonists alone. Studies showed that ipratropium produces a significant additional increase in forced expiratory volume at 1 second (FEV$_1$) above that achieved with albuterol alone. Studies found a significantly greater improvement in FEV$_1$ with ipratropium and albuterol compared with albuterol alone when given at the onset of therapy. As more experience with the use of ipratropium accumulates, its niche in the treatment of acute asthma will become clearer; the available data seem to support its consideration for moderately to severely ill patients. Glycopyrrolate (Robinul) is another anticholinergic agent available in aerosolized form that may be effective in treating acute asthma exacerbations.

### Magnesium Sulfate and Other Drugs

Studies assessing the use of intravenous magnesium sulfate for the treatment of status asthmaticus in adults have had mixed results. In one report, four pediatric patients with severe asthma demonstrated an apparent benefit with no adverse effects when doses of 40 to 50 mg/kg were infused over 20 minutes. Another study found a significant improvement in short-term pulmonary function in children aged 6 to 18 years with moderate to severe asthma when they were treated with intravenous magnesium sulfate given at a dose of 25 mg/kg. Clear documentation of objective improvement with the use of magnesium sulfate has been difficult because of the lack of control groups and the concurrent use of other bronchodilators. Magnesium sulfate may be useful in treating a subset of children with asthma. Similarly, currently available calcium channel blockers do not have a clinically significant bronchodilating effect, but newer agents are being developed. Leukotriene antagonists, lipooxygenase inhibitors, nitric acid donors, and potassium channel openers are in investigational stages.

## Patient Management

Based on the initial history, physical examination, and laboratory assessments, patients should be stratified by severity of illness. Of course, during the ED stay the degree of illness may change, so that frequent examinations to assess response to therapy are critically important. This categorization, however, will help ensure that appropriately aggressive therapy is administered to the most severely ill patients and will provide a starting point from which management can begin.

### Mild Exacerbation

A mild exacerbation is characterized by alertness, slight tachycardia, expiratory wheezing only, minimal accessory muscle use, an inspiratory-to-expiratory ratio of 1:1, and an oxygen saturation greater than 97%. For such children,

---

### ED MANAGEMENT OF ACUTE EXACERBATIONS OF ASTHMA IN CHILDREN

**INITIAL TREATMENT**

- Oxygen to keep saturation >95%
- Nebulized Ventolin (albuterol), 0.5 mg/kg/dose (maximum, 5 mg/dose) or Ventolin metered dose inhaler every 20 minutes as needed up to three treatments
- Subcutaneous epinephrine, 0.01 mg/kg (0.01 mL/kg of 1:1000 solution; maximum, 0.3 mg/dose) every 20 minutes as needed up to three treatments for any child who has a decreased level of consciousness, or if a child 5 years of age or older is unable to generate a peak expiratory flow rate (PEFR)
- If the child has no response after one nebulized treatment or is steroid dependent, administer one of the following steroids:
  1. Oral prednisone or oral methylprednisolone, 1–2 mg/kg/dose
  2. Intravenous methylprednisolone, 1–2 mg/kg/dose
  3. Inhaled dexamethasone, 1.5 mg/kg

#### EVALUATION AND TREATMENT AFTER 1 HOUR OR THREE TREATMENTS

| Good Response | Incomplete Response | Poor Response |
|---|---|---|
| - Normalization of vital signs<br>- Normal level of consciousness for age<br>- $O_2$ saturation $\geq$ 95% on room air<br>- Minimal absent signs of respiratory distress<br>- PEFR $\geq$ 80% of normal baseline | - Increased heart and respiratory rate<br>- Normal level of consciousness for age<br>- $O_2$ saturation 90%–94% on room air<br>- Moderate signs of respiratory distress<br>- PEFR 50%–80% of normal baseline | - Increased heart and respiratory rate<br>- Decrease in level of consciousness<br>- $O_2$ saturation < 90% on room air<br>- Decreased air movement and severe accessory muscle use<br>- PEFR < 50% of normal baseline |
| ↓ | ↓ | ↓ |
| - Discharge to home with patient education regarding avoiding asthma triggers, administering medications, and follow-up visit | - Continue nebulized ß₂-agonist treatments every 20 minutes or as a continuous aerosol<br>- Nebulized ipratropium bromide, 250 µg/kg, or nebulized glucopyrrolate, 1 mg<br>- Magnesium sulfate, 40–50 mg/kg intravenously over 30 minutes<br>- Consider inpatient admission if no improvement of respiratory distress is noted<br>- If improvement, discharge to home with patient education | - Admit to hospital<br>- Consider continuous ß₂-agonist nebulization, intravenous steroids, and anticholinergic therapy |

Source: Tom Stein, MD, FACEP, and Richard Scarfone, MD, "Management of Acute Asthma in Children," *Topics in Emergency Medicine,* Vol. 18:3, Aspen Publishers, Inc., © September 1996.

albuterol should be administered by nebulization in 100% oxygen at a rate of 6 to 8 L/min. Patients should be reassessed frequently, and albuterol may be repeated every 20 to 30 minutes as needed.

A subset of children with an initially mild exacerbation will experience clinical deterioration, which is an indication for more aggressive therapy (see below). The majority of others, however, will respond promptly to the above therapy and will be well enough to be discharged home after two or three nebulizations. These children should be sent home with a 7-day course of either oral or inhaled albuterol, which can then be used as needed for wheezing beyond that time. In addition, a 5-day course of oral prednisone is indicated for children who were already receiving daily ß$_2$-agonists on arrival to the ED, who had a poor response to albuterol, or who have a history of frequent ED visits or hospitalizations for asthma.

## Moderate Exacerbation

Children who are alert but tachypneic with inspiratory and expiratory wheezing, significant accessory muscle use, an inspiratory-to-expiratory ratio of 1:2, and an oxygen saturation of 92% to 97% are experiencing a moderate attack. Nebulized albuterol should be administered promptly, and supplemental oxygen should be provided if the initial oxygen saturation is 95% or less in room air. Corticosteroids should be administered immediately after the initial albuterol treatment. For patients who have been vomiting at home before the ED visit or who vomit the oral prednisone, parenteral steroids should be administered.

Albuterol treatments should be continued every 20 to 30 minutes, with clinical reassessment preceding each nebulization. The clinician should use the patient's clinical response in determining the duration of ED therapy and disposition. Those patients who show prompt improvement soon after ED arrival may be discharged home. It is wise to delay a disposition decision until 30 to 40 minutes after the most recent albuterol treatment so that the clinical relapse can be noted. Albuterol and corticosteroids should be prescribed for all such patients, as described earlier. On the other hand, 90 minutes after arrival in the ED, most children will have received three or four albuterol treatments. When subjective and objective measures reveal that the degree of respiratory distress is unchanged at this point, hospitalization is warranted.

Clinicians can have the greatest impact on that subset of moderately ill children who experience some clinical improvement after three or four albuterol nebulizations and steroid treatment but are not well enough to be sent home. Treatment of such children with albuterol every 30 minutes for a total of 3 to 4 hours may allow outpatient management. One study showed that, among prednisone-treated children

who would have been hospitalized after 2 hours of ED therapy, fewer than half were actually hospitalized when aggressive ß$_2$-agonist therapy was continued for an additional 2 hours. Presumably, the onset of prednisone's effects allowed these children to avoid hospitalization.

## Severe Exacerbation

A severe exacerbation is characterized by restlessness or lethargy, extreme tachypnea, wheezing that is audible without a stethoscope, significant use of accessory muscles, an inspiratory-to-expiratory ratio above 1:2, and an oxygen saturation greater than 92%. Some children with a severe exacerbation may have a slowed respiratory rate because of a prolonged expiratory phase, and wheezing may not be audible if aeration is markedly decreased.

Continuous monitoring of heart and respiratory rate, pulse oximetry, and blood pressure should be performed. Supplying oxygen and promptly administering a ß$_2$-agonist are the initial steps to take in the treatment of severely ill children. To achieve an oxygen saturation of 95% or greater, it may be necessary to employ a non-rebreathing face mask. An intravenous line should be established as soon as possible and methylprednisolone administered. For children with poor inspiratory flow, albuterol is not effectively delivered to the small airways; subcutaneous terbutaline or epinephrine may be used in this setting. Others will benefit from albuterol delivered by continuous nebulization. Alternatively, a ß$_2$-agonist may be administered as a continuous intravenous infusion. For severely ill children, arterial blood gas measurement will be helpful to determine the adequacy of ventilation. Many of these children will require admission to the hospital's intensive care unit for close observation and management.

## A SYSTEMS APPROACH TO ASTHMA CARE*

The main goal in managing asthma is presenting acute exacerbations and providing early treatment for those that occur. Experts suggest that the major factors contributing to morbidity and mortality associated with asthma are underdiagnosis and inappropriate treatment. Many hospitalizations are preventable since they are due to a failure in outpatient management.

In September 1994, Principal Health Care of Louisiana (PHCLa) launched an intervention to improve the care of children with asthma. PHCLa is a 26,600-member independent practice association (IPA) model health maintenance

*Source: Thomas F. Plaut et al., "A Systems Approach to Asthma Care," *Managed Care Quarterly,* Vol. 4:3, Aspen Publishers, Inc., © Summer 1996.

organization (HMO) managed by Principal Health Care with headquarters in Rockville, Maryland. Forty-six pediatricians, 13 in solo practice and 33 in seven pediatric groups, care for Principal's 6,642 members under age 15. Principal's members account for only 1 to 25 percent of each physician's patient load. Of the 18 HMOs managed by Principal Health Care, the Louisiana plan had the highest hospitalization rate for childhood asthma. In 1993, asthma generated 9.6 hospital days per 1,000 PHCLa child enrollees, or 101 percent of the U.S. rate for 1993. The admission rate was 3.5 per 1,000, or 125 percent of the U.S. rate. Cost for hospitalizations was $82,734, averaging $1,293 per day (Table 1).

Plan managers identified pediatric asthma as a likely area for improving care and saving costs if hospitalizations could be reduced. After a feasibility study confirmed this view, Principal administrators agreed that a comprehensive program could be cost-effective. A physician consultant then analyzed PHCLa baseline hospitalization data for 1993 using the HMO Data Sheet (Table 2). An improvement in outpatient asthma care could reduce hospital days for asthma by 33 percent during the first year of the intervention, and half that amount during the second year. This effort could lower the Principal rate for asthma hospital days to 50 percent of the national rate for 1993 and could save a total of 53 days during a two-year intervention from September 1, 1994 to August 31, 1996.

The intervention focuses on provider education emphasizing early diagnosis of asthma, early use of oral steroids, proper use of inhalation devices, objective monitoring of patient status, and use of daily preventive treatment. Patient education is an integral part of treatment. This approach

**Table 2.** HMO Data Sheet

Number of child enrollees under 15 years of age on January 1, 1993: 7,671
Number of child enrollees under 15 years of age on January 1, 1994: 5,613

**Average for 1993 is 6,642.**

Hospitalizations under 15 years of age after newborn discharge in 1993:

| | New Orleans | | | U.S. 1993 |
|---|---|---|---|---|
| | Discharges | Days | Rate per 1,000 | Rate per 1,000 |
| Asthma (ICD CM-9 493) | 23 | 64 | 9.6 | 9.5 |
| Acute Bronchitis/ Bronchiolitis (ICD CM-9 466) | 5 | 14 | 2.1 | N.A. |
| Pneumonia (ICD CM-9 480–486) | 15 | 63 | 9.5 | 12.6 |

supports the primary care physician as the provider and coordinator of care by supplying monitoring and treatment devices, books, diaries, home care services, and allergy consultation. It also manifests a systems approach to asthma care in its reliance on a nurse case manager who oversees patient and family support networks.

## Specific Intervention Activities

Managers accepted the physician consultant's stipulation that every admission for asthma should be considered due to failure of outpatient treatment unless proven otherwise. Patients were not to be blamed for poor asthma control.

Primary care physicians are the cornerstone of this intervention. They initiate and manage all aspects of patient care. Six asthma advocates—three pediatricians, an internist, and two allergists—were selected by the health services manager because of their interest in asthma, their good working relationships with Principal, and their membership in major practice groups. They maintain continuous dialogue with the physician consultant and communicate current asthma care practices to their colleagues.

Through this intervention the physicians can offer a broad array of essential resources at no cost to the patient: durable medical equipment (e.g., compressor-driven nebulizers, peak flow meters and holding chambers); a home care program for assessment, education, and skill building; and consultation with an allergist (see box entitled "Resources for Primary Care Practitioners"). Principal provides a copy of the 40-page basic asthma guide, *One Minute Asthma: What You*

**Table 1.** Baseline Data for Principal Health Care, New Orleans 1993

| | |
|---|---|
| Membership in IPA/HMO | 26,656 |
| Pediatric membership | 6,642 |
| Pediatric membership as a % of total | 24.9% |
| Number of children with asthma | 482 |
| Prevalence of asthma in children | 7.25% |
| Pediatric hospital days 1993 | 64 |

Goal: Reduce hospital stays for childhood asthma by 33% from baseline in first year and 50% in second year, a total reduction of 53 days.

| | |
|---|---|
| Average hospital cost per day | $ 1,293 |
| Expected savings (53 × $1,293) | 68,529 |
| Costs: | |
| Physician Consultant | 18,000 |
| Consultant travel and travel time | 6,500 |
| Equipment and books | 8,502 |
| Projected net saving: | 35,527 |

### Resources for Primary Care Practitioners

Home care services
Consultation with allergist
Equipment
    Peak flow meters
    Holding chambers
    Compressor-driven nebulizers
Literature
    *One Minute Asthma: What You Need To Know*
    *Children with Asthma: A Manual for Parents*
    Asthma diaries and matching home treatment plans
Phone contact with consultant

*Need To Know,* to the family of each asthma patient. A more comprehensive book, *Children with Asthma: A Manual for Parents,* is given to families whose children have moderate or severe asthma problems. Estimated costs for equipment and books are listed in Table 3. Patients are managed through the entire continuum of care in a manner consistent with the National Heart, Lung, and Blood Institute (NHLBI) *Guidelines for the Diagnosis and Management of Asthma.*

A two-day site visit by the physician consultant in September 1994 included two conferences for 80 physicians, office nurses, school nurses, and respiratory therapists. Two additional conferences were held in March 1995 during the second site visit. Each of these conferences emphasized six basic points:

1. the early diagnosis of asthma
2. early use of steroids
3. proper use of inhalation devices
4. objective monitoring of the patient's status
5. use of preventive medicines for asthma
6. the use of uniform educational material and treatment plans.

These points are emphasized throughout the consultant's conferences and visits, and in educational materials provided to physicians. They are also presented in the books, diaries, and home treatment plans used by home care staff, as well as in the allergists' consultations.

Many physicians hold outdated beliefs that can hinder the implementation of this program. To address these issues, the physician consultant stated these beliefs, the corresponding facts, and their potential solutions in his meetings with physicians.

## Early Diagnosis of Asthma

**Belief:** The diagnosis of asthma will frighten and upset parents.

**Fact:** Absence of the diagnosis will deprive parents or patients of the opportunity to learn about asthma and to intervene early in the course of an attack.

**Solution:** Describe asthma as an illness with a broad range of severity. Parents will be reassured to hear that most cases are mild.

## Early Use of Oral Steroids

**Belief:** Overuse may cause serious side effects.

**Fact:** Oral steroids are the most potent medicine available to treat inflammation during an attack. Concern with overuse leads to underuse: thus many patients who would benefit from oral steroids do not get them. As a result, they will require emergency care or admission to the hospital where they will receive high doses of steroids.

**Table 3.** Cost Estimate for Equipment and Books per 1,000 Child Enrollees

| Equipment or book | Distribution (%) | Number needed | Cost per item | Total cost per 1,000 enrollees |
|---|---|---|---|---|
| Peak flow meter | 60 | 30 | $20.00 | $600 |
| Compressor-driven nebulizer | 30 | 15 | 65.00 | 975 |
| Holding chamber | 70 | 35 | 20.00 | 700 |
| *One Minute Asthma* | 100 | 50 | 1.50 | 75 |
| *Children with Asthma* | 40 | 20 | 4.25 | 85 |
| Asthma diaries (pads of 100) | 100 | 12.5 | 10.0 | 125 |
| **TOTAL (two years)** | | | | **$2,560** |

This estimate assumes 5 percent of children in the plan have asthma. The 6,642 enrollees will need $17,004 worth of equipment and books. Since half of these materials would have been purchased without the intervention, the charge to the intervention is $8,502.

**Solution:** Describe the 1988 study that shows early use of steroids decreased hospitalizations by 90 percent in an experimental group. Because these patients had fewer serious episodes, they used less steroids than the control group.

## Use of Inhalation Devices

Compressor-driven nebulizer:

**Belief:** Home administration of an adrenaline-like medicine by compressor-driven nebulizer is dangerous because a parent might treat too often and cause toxicity.

**Fact:** The major danger of using the compressor-driven nebulizer at home is that it can mask symptoms. An inadequately instructed patient or parent will not recognize that the asthma is going out of control.

**Solution:** Give patients a home treatment plan based on the asthma care zones as determined by peak flow or asthma signs. This will limit the frequency of use and will direct parents at what point to see the doctor.

Holding chamber:

**Belief:** Most patients who use metered-dose inhalers (MDIs) will not benefit from using a holding chamber.

**Fact:** The holding chamber increases the benefits of inhaled steroids and decreases the side effects of all medicines delivered by MDI.

**Solution:** Ask physician to demonstrate proper MDI use with and without holding chamber during hands-on practice. The physician will appreciate the difficulty patients have in using the MDI alone and the ease of its use with a holding chamber.

## Objective Monitoring of Patient Status

Monitoring peak flow:

**Belief:** An asthma symptom diary is just as good as a peak flow diary in helping patients manage asthma.

**Fact:** Peak flow often drops before symptoms occur. The peak flow meter is the best tool for assessing asthma at home.

**Solution:** The Asthma Peak Flow Diary, which includes both peak flow scores and symptoms, can serve as an educational, monitoring, and management tool for patients over four years of age (see "Sample Asthma Peak Flow Diary").

Monitoring asthma signs:

**Belief:** Parents are not competent to assess asthma symptoms in children under five.

**Fact:** Well-trained parents can accurately assess their child's status.

**Solution:** Provide asthma assessment system based on signs that parents can hear and see, using the Asthma Signs Diary (see "Sample Asthma Signs Diary").

## Daily Preventive Treatment

**Belief:** Only about 10 percent of asthma patients need to take preventive medicine daily.

**Fact:** About 40 percent of asthma patients, practically all of those with symptoms more than two days per week, will benefit from daily preventive medicine.

**Solution:** Encourage physicians to prescribe preventive treatment for their patients with moderate asthma while tracking them with an asthma diary. They will be impressed with the results.

## Education

**Belief:** Prescribing medicines is much more important than providing asthma education.

**Fact:** Many asthma patients take their medicines improperly and derive little benefit from them. Patients who do not understand what triggers their asthma attacks cannot prevent them.

**Solution:** Teach doctors the correct techniques for taking medicines and ways that patients can avoid their asthma triggers.

This asthma intervention is grounded in the care provided by primary care physicians and other clinical managers. At PHCLa, the essential starting point was the actions of the PHCLa health services manager, who initiated the asthma intervention and coordinated each step of the process with the various participants, including the physician consultant, nurse case manager, medical director, and the asthma advocates. Specifically, the health services manager:

- evaluated and hired the consultant
- designed a process that led to adoption of the NHLBI *Guidelines* for Principal Health Care physicians
- selected six asthma advocates
- expanded the original program to include allergy consultation and home care services
- adopted criteria for referral to an allergist (see box entitled "Criteria for Allergy Referral") and determined proper source of compensation
- decided on home care treatment guidelines and services needed and hired a vendor (see box entitled "Home Care Visit Plan")
- broadened the scope of intervention to include adults and selected seven additional asthma advocates.

The asthma intervention is committed to case management. The plan's nurse case manager is the liaison between the health services manager, the physician consultant, and

# SAMPLE ASTHMA PEAK FLOW DIARY

**Name:** *Jane Doe*
See back for instructions.

## ASTHMA DIARY PEAK FLOW

*Please bring to each visit.*

O - Before bronchodilator
X - After bronchodilator

### Peak Flow Rate

| Zone | % | Value |
|---|---|---|
| Green Zone | 100% | 200 |
| High Yellow Zone | 80% | 160 |
| Low Yellow Zone | 65% | 130 |
| Red Zone | 50% | 100 |

### Medicines*

| Medicine | Dose | 12/8 | 12/9 | 12/10 | 12/11 | 12/12 | 12/13 | 12/14 | 12/15 | 12/16 | 12/17 | 12/18 |
|---|---|---|---|---|---|---|---|---|---|---|---|---|
| Intal - 2 ampules Cromolyn or Nedocromil | 2x | | | | | | | | | | | |
| Inhaled steroid | | √√√ | √√√ | √√√ | √√√ | √√√ | √√√ | √√√ | √√√ | √√√ | √√√ | √√√ |
| Ventolin - 0.5 cc Albuterol | 2 - 6 x | √ | √ | √ | √√ | √√√ | √√√ | √√√ | √√√ | √√√ | √√√ | √√√ |
| Prelone 1½ t. Oral steroid | 1x | √ | √ | √ | √ | √ | √ | √ | √ | | | |
| Theophylline | | | | | | | | | | | | |

### Signs

| Sign | 12/8 | 12/9 | 12/10 | 12/11 | 12/12 | 12/13 | 12/14 | 12/15 | 12/16 | 12/17 | 12/18 |
|---|---|---|---|---|---|---|---|---|---|---|---|
| Wheeze | 1 | 0 | 0 | 1 | | | | | | | |
| Cough | 1 | 1 | 1 | 1 | | | | | | | |
| Activity | 0 | 0 | 0 | 0 | | | | | | | |
| Sleep | 1 | 0 | 0 | 0 | | | | | | | |

**Triggers, Comments:**
12/8 — (blank)
12/9 — (blank)
12/10 — Has cold
12/11 — Feels better
12/12 — More active
12/13 — Cough - cold air
12/14 — Stomach ache
12/15 — Stomach ache
12/16 — Very tired

## Signs

◆ **Wheeze:**
None .............................. 0
Exhale only ................... 1
Throughout entire
exhale ............................ 2
Both inhale and exhale ... 3

◆ **Cough:**
None .............................. 0
Less than one
per minute ..................... 1
One to four per minute ... 2
More than four
per minute ..................... 3

◆ **Activity:**
Fully active .................... 0
Can run short distance .... 1
Can walk only
Missed school or
stayed indoors ............... 3

◆ **Sleep:**
Fine ............................... 0
Slight wheeze or
cough ............................. 1
Awake 2-3 times,
wheeze or cough ............ 2
Awake most of
the time .......................... 3

**Books available from Pedipress (800-344-5864):**
• *Children with Asthma: A Manual for Parents*
• *One Minute Asthma: What You Need to Know*
• *El asma en un minuto*
• *Winning Over Asthma*
• *Asthma Charts & Forms for the Physician's Office*

*Medicines: • Cromolyn (*Intal*) • Nedocromil (*Tilade*) • Inhaled steroid (*AeroBid, Azmacort, Beclovent, Vanceril*) • Albuterol (*Proventil, Ventolin*) • Oral steroid (*prednisone, Prelone, Pediapred*) • Theophylline (*Slo-bid capsules, Theo-Dur tablets*). Your doctor may prescribe others.

## SAMPLE ASTHMA SIGNS DIARY

**Name:** John Doe
See back for instructions.

### ASTHMA DIARY SIGNS

*Please bring to each visit.*

Before bronchodilator-O
After bronchodilator-X

| Signs | Date | 4/1 | 4/2 | 4/3 | 4/3 | 4/4 | 4/4 | 4/5 | 4/5 | 4/6 | 4/6 | 4/7 | 4/7 | 4/8 | 4/9 |
|---|---|---|---|---|---|---|---|---|---|---|---|---|---|---|---|
| | Triggers, Comments | Good day | | Husky | Slightly husky | | | | | Very irritable | | Visit with doctor | | | |
| Cough | | 0 0 | 0 1 | 1 1 | 2 1 | 2 1 | 2 2 | 2 1 | 2 1 | 1 1 | 2 1 | 1 0 | 0 0 | 0 1 | 0 0 |
| Wheeze | | 0 0 | 0 0 | 1 1 | 2 1 | 2 1 | 2 1 | 2 1 | 2 1 | 2 0 | 2 1 | 1 0 | 0 0 | 0 0 | 0 0 |
| Chest skin | | 0 0 | 0 0 | 0 0 | 0 0 | 0 0 | 0 0 | 0 0 | 0 0 | 0 0 | 0 0 | 0 0 | 0 0 | 0 0 | 0 0 |
| Breathing faster | | 0 0 | 0 0 | 1 0 | 2 1 | 1 1 | 1 1 | 1 1 | 1 1 | 1 0 | 1 0 | 0 0 | 0 0 | 0 0 | 0 0 |
| **TOTAL:** | | 0 0 | 1 0 | 3 2 | 6 3 | 5 4 | 5 4 | 5 3 | 4 2 | 4 1 | 3 2 | 2 0 | 0 0 | 1 0 | 0 0 |

**Zones**

| | 0 | Green Zone |
| 1 | |
| 2 | High Yellow Zone |
| 3 | |
| 4 | |
| 5 | |
| 6 | Low Yellow Zone |
| 7 | |
| 8 | |
| 9 | Red Zone |

**Medicines***

| Medicine | 4/1 | 4/2 | 4/3 | 4/3 | 4/4 | 4/4 | 4/5 | 4/5 | 4/6 | 4/6 | 4/7 | 4/7 | 4/8 | 4/9 |
|---|---|---|---|---|---|---|---|---|---|---|---|---|---|---|
| Intal - 2 ampules Cromolyn 2x | ✓✓ | ✓✓ | ✓✓ | ✓ | ✓ | ✓ | ✓ | ✓ | ✓ | ✓ | ✓ | ✓ | ✓ | ✓ |
| Proventil- Ambuterol 0.25 ml | ✓✓ | ✓✓ | ✓✓ | ✓✓ | ✓✓ | ✓✓ | ✓✓ | ✓ | ✓ | ✓ | ✓ | ✓✓ | ✓✓ | ✓✓ |
| Prelone Oral steroid 4 mL 1 dose | | | | ✓ | ✓ | ✓ | ✓ | ✓ | | | | | | |
| Theophylline | | | | | | | | | | | | | | |

**Daily**

| | 4/1 | 4/2 | 4/3 | 4/3 | 4/4 | 4/4 | 4/5 | 4/5 | 4/6 | 4/6 | 4/7 | 4/7 | 4/8 | 4/9 |
|---|---|---|---|---|---|---|---|---|---|---|---|---|---|---|
| Activity | 0 | 0 | 1 | 1 | 1 | 1 | 1 | 1 | 1 | 0 | 0 | 1 | 1 | |
| Sleep | 0 | 0 | 0 | 1 | 1 | 0 | 0 | 0 | 0 | 0 | 1 | 0 | | |

### Signs

♦ **Cough in past hour:**
None . . . . . . . . . 0
Less than one per minute . . . . . 1
1-4 per minute . . . . . 2
More than four per minute . . . . . 3

♦ **Wheeze:**
None . . . . . . . . . 0
Barely noticeable . . . . 1
Full exhale . . . . . 2
Inhale & exhale . . . . 3

♦ **Sucking in chest skin:**
None . . . . . . . . . 0
Barely noticeable . . . . 1
Obvious . . . . . . . 2
Severe . . . . . . . . 3

♦ **Breathing faster:**
None . . . . . . . . . 0
Slight increase . . . . . 1
Up to 50% increase . . . 2
Over 50% increase . . . . 3

### Daily Routine

♦ **Activity**
Usual . . . . . . . . . 0
Walking less . . . . . . 1
Plays quietly . . . . . . 2
Sleeping during day . . . . 3

♦ **Sleep:**
Fine . . . . . . . . . 0
Slight wheeze or cough . . . . 1
Awake 2-3 times because of wheeze or cough . . . . . 2
Awake most of the time . . . . 3

*MEDICINES: Cromolyn (*Intal*); Albuterol (*Proventil, Ventolin*); Oral steroid (*prednisone, Prelone, Pediapred*); Theophylline (*Slo-bid capsules*); Your doctor may prescribe others.

## Criteria for Allergy Referral

Consider specialty referral if:

- Patient is not responding optimally to the asthma therapy after three office visits
- Patient requires guidance on environmental control, consideration of immunotherapy, smoking cessation, complications of therapy, or difficult compliance issues
- Clinical entities complicate airway disease (e.g., sinusitis, nasal polyps, aspergillosis, and severe rhinitis); or
- Patient has had a life-threatening acute asthma exacerbation, has poor self-management ability, or has difficult family dynamics.

Source: From Care Guideline, Asthma in Children (revised December 1993). Institute for Clinical Systems Integration, One Appletree Square, Suite 1155, 8009 34th Avenue South, Bloomington, MN 55425. Used with permission.

## Home Care Visit Plan

First visit, within one day of discharge from hospital (except weekends)
- Observation/physical assessment.
- Initial home assessment and history for possible triggers.
- Brief explanation of asthma (give *One Minute Asthma* booklet).
- Medication review and teaching including return demonstration of inhaler/spacer (Aerochamber)/compressor-driven nebulizer (ProNeb).
- Review red zone signs and plan.
- Discuss follow-up visits/when to call doctor.

Second visit
- Observation/physical assessment.
- Complete asthma teaching, give home treatment plan based on age.
- Introduce instructions on how to use a peak flow meter/introduce Asthma Peak Flow Diary.
- Return demonstration of compressor-driven nebulizer/holding chamber/inhaler.
- Completion of home assessment/instruct on how to avoid or eliminate trigger factors.
- Verify physician follow-up/discuss plan for school setting.

Third visit
- Observation/physical assessment.
- Evaluation of understanding and compliance.
- Review asthma peak flow meter use.
- Review and reinforce physician's instructions.
- Discharge instructions/review when to seek appropriate medication intervention.

Source: Asthma Program Home Visit Protocol, developed for Principal Health Care for Pediatric Services of America, 3159 Campus Drive, Norcross, Georgia 30071. Used with permission.

the other participants and is the key staff person during the implementation phase of the intervention. The case manager's responsibilities include:

Preparation for conferences
—discusses materials needed with consultant
—sends literature out inviting to the conference 180 primary care physicians, emergency room physicians and staff, allergists and pulmonologists who care for PHCLa patients as well as local school nurses
—obtains commitment to attend from physicians
—arranges facilities for meetings.
Interactions with health services manager:
—meets to review each asthma hospitalization
—reports on performance of home care vendors
—alerts health services manager if problems occur with services in hospital, emergency room, or physician's office.
Interactions with consultant:
—provides asthma hospitalization data on a regular basis
—provides additional information on various aspects of the program.
Interactions with patients:
—sees each patient in the hospital to track status and treatment
—informally assesses patient satisfaction with program.

The physician consultant advised the plan with respect to the content, approach, and sequence of the intervention, as well as the purchase of equipment and books.

During the first year, the consultant will spent the equivalent of 12 days on the project: two two-day visits and eight days of preparation and follow-up by letter, fax, and phone. The second year, the consultant will make one two-day site visit and spend four days following up by letter and phone. Though primary care physicians almost always use the consultation services of Principal Health Care allergists in New Orleans, they are free to contact the program's physician consultant at any time with a patient or intervention-related question.

In addition to the books, home treatment plans were recommended based on peak flow (see "Peak Flow–Based Treatment Plan") and asthma signs (see "Signs-Based Home Treatment Plan"), which dovetail with the diaries. Together these materials allow physicians, home care staff, and family to provide a consistent approach to care.

A three-visit home care program is recommended for each patient after hospital discharge and, in some cases, after a visit to the emergency room. This program includes a patient and home assessment, basic asthma education, and review of medicines, delivery devices, and peak flow monitoring. Home management is based on the asthma diaries and home treatment plans.

In the first nine months of the PHCLa intervention, the following steps were taken and results noted:

- 1993 Principal rate of hospital stays for asthma was 9.6 per 1,000 members, or 101 percent of the 1993 U.S. rate (9.5 per 1,000), a total of 64 days for children under 15.
- Summer 1994: Consultant reviews Principal's hospitalization data. Based on previous interventions, he believes asthma hospitalization could be reduced by 50 percent during a two-year intervention.
- September 1994: Intervention begins. Asthma advocates are selected. First on-site consultation and conferences for physicians and other health professionals are held. Consultant visits practice sites of the six asthma advocates.
- November 1994: Criteria for allergy referrals are established and home care program is initiated.
- March 1995: Second on-site consultation is held with family practitioners, internists, and pediatricians totaling 90 physicians. Adult care asthma advocates selected in preparation for expansion of the intervention to adults.
- April 1995: Addition of adult patients quadruples size of the intervention population and more than triples the number of primary care physicians.

## Data Collection and Analysis

In order for a health plan to compare its data across sites and programs with accuracy, it must use identical definitions and demographic criteria.

*Data.* Hospital days and admission/discharge data should be collected automatically by the financial planning and analysis department in the corporate office. Data should also be collected locally as a control.

*Age range.* National Center for Health Statistics data show that the younger the child, the higher the admission rate for asthma. This intervention includes children from newborn discharge to the 15th birthday. A similar program that ex-cludes infants or includes teenagers after their 15th birthday will have a lower discharge rate.

*Hospital days versus discharges.* Hospital days are a better indicator of the care children receive for asthma than hospital discharges. They distinguish between the child who needs short rescue therapy and a child whose poor outpatient management necessitates a prolonged stay. They also are not confounded by transfer from one hospital to another.

*Diagnosis of asthma.* Misdiagnosis has been recognized as a problem since 1978, and physicians were urged to diagnose asthma in most patients they had previously labeled as having bronchitis, wheezy bronchitis, or bronchospasm. In addition, asthma was recognized as the major cause of recurrent pneumonia in 1982. It is likely that 100,000 of the 300,000 children hospitalized for bronchitis, bronchiolitis, and pneumonia in 1988 should have been diagnosed with asthma. If asthma is not diagnosed, it cannot be treated optimally.

*Diagnostic transfer.* Hospital days for asthma are the major outcome measure for this intervention. However, PHCLa monitored and analyzed asthma hospital admissions and collected data for pneumonia, bronchitis, and bronchiolitis to achieve a fuller understanding of results. The misdiagnosis of asthma as pneumonia or bronchitis is a common problem, particularly in children under five years of age, and can skew data positively or negatively. For example, physicians who improve their diagnostic ability will shift a diagnosis from pneumonia to asthma, worsening their asthma statistics. Conversely, physicians who want to improve their asthma statistics might shift a diagnosis from asthma to pneumonia. Finally, an epidemic of viral pneumonia might lead to a rise in rates for asthma, as well as bronchitis, bronchiolitis, and pneumonia.

*Emergency room.* The PHCLa intervention has not yet reviewed data on patient visits to the emergency room. Data will be monitored to see whether emergency visits increase as hospital days decrease.

## Implementation Issues

Consistency is an essential component of any asthma intervention, and educational materials help ensure a true systems approach at PHCLa. The NHLBI *Guidelines* provides clear protocols for the important aspects of patient care. After PHCLa adopted them, the *Guidelines* became the common basis for the plan's discussion of asthma care. All the primary care physicians use the same books, monitoring tools, and medical equipment, and refer patients to allergists and home care providers who use them as well. Thus, patients receive a consistent message that uses the same words, whether coming from their regular physician, on-call physician, consulting allergist, home care staff, or emergency room physician, and from all educational materials.

# For Adults, Teens, and Children Age 5 and Over: Peak Flow–Based Home Treatment Plan

Name: _____    Date: _____    Best Peak Flow: _____

**GREEN ZONE: Peak flow between _____ and _____.**
- **Normal activity.**
  - ☐ *Albuterol (Proventil, Ventolin):* 1 or 2 puffs 15 minutes before exercise.
  - ☐ *Cromolyn (Intal):* 2 puffs before contact with cat or other allergen.
- **Medicine to be taken every day:**
  - ☐ *Nedocromil (Tilade)* or *cromolyn (Intal):* ___ puffs ___ times a day (a total of ____ puffs daily).
  - ☐ *Inhaled steroid* (Aerobid, Azmacort, Beclovent, Vanceril): ____ puffs ____ times a day (a total of ____ puffs daily).
  - ☐ *Albuterol (Proventil, Ventolin):* ____ puffs before each *nedocromil, cromolyn,* or *inhaled steroid* dose for the first month.
  - ☐ *Theophylline* (Slo-bid capsules, Theo-Dur tablets): ___ mg ___ times a day (a total of ___ mg daily).

**HIGH YELLOW ZONE: Peak flow between _____ and _____.**
- **Eliminate triggers and change medicines. No strenuous exercise.**
- **Medicine to be taken:**
  - ✓ *Albuterol:* ____ puffs by holding chamber. Give three to six times in 24 hours. Continue until peak flow is in the *Green Zone* for two days.
  - ✓ Double *inhaled steroid* to ___ puffs daily until peak flow is in the *Green Zone* for as long as it was in the *Yellow Zone.*

- - - - - - - - - - - - - - - - - - - - - - - - - - - - - - - - - - - - - - - -

**LOW YELLOW ZONE: Peak flow between _____ and _____.**
Follow this plan if peak flow does not reach *High Yellow Zone* within 10 minutes after taking inhaled *albuterol,* or drops back into *Low Yellow Zone* within four hours:
- ✓ Continue albuterol treatment as above.
- ✓ Add *oral steroid*\* ____ mg immediately. Continue each morning (8:00 AM) until peak flow is in the *Green Zone* for at least 24 hours.

\*If your condition does not improve within two days after starting oral steroid, or if peak flow does not reach the *green zone* within seven days of treatment, see your doctor.

**RED ZONE: Peak flow less than _____.**
Follow this plan if peak flow does not reach *Low Yellow Zone* within 10 minutes after taking inhaled *albuterol,* or drops back into *Red Zone* within four hours:
- ✓ *Albuterol* ____ puffs by holding chamber.
- ✓ **Give *oral steroid* ____ mg.**
- ✓ **Visit your doctor.**

# For Children under Age 5:
# Signs–Based Home Treatment Plan

Name:                                                          Date:

### Green Zone

**GREEN ZONE: Absolutely no cough, wheeze, breathing faster, or sucking in of the chest skin.**
- **Normal activity.**
- **Medicine to be taken every day:**
  - ☐ *Cromolyn (Intal):* ____ ampules in ____ doses.
  - ☐ *Albuterol (Proventil, Ventolin):* ____ cc by compressor-driven nebulizer with each *cromolyn* dose for the first month.
  - ☐ *Theophylline* (Slo-bid capsules): ____ mg ____ times a day (a total of ____ mg daily).

### Yellow Zone

**HIGH YELLOW ZONE: Total asthma sign score 1 to 4 measured before taking inhaled bronchodilator.**
- **Eliminate triggers and change medicines.**
- **Medicine to be taken:**
  - ✓ *Cromolyn:* as above.
  - ✓ *Albuterol:* 0.__ cc in 2 cc *cromolyn* or saline by compressor-driven nebulizer. Give three to six times in 24 hours. Continue until signs score is 0 or 1 for 48 hours.

- - - - - - - - - - - - - - - - - - - - - - - - - - - - - - - - - - - - - - - - - -

**LOW YELLOW ZONE: Total asthma sign score 5 to 8.**

**Follow this plan if sign score does not reach *High Yellow Zone* within 10 minutes after taking inhaled *albuterol*, or drops back into *Low Yellow Zone* within four hours:**
- **No strenuous exercise.**
- **Medicine to be taken:**
  - ✓ Continue *albuterol and cromolyn* as above.
  - ✓ Start *oral steroid* * ____ mg, ____ cc immediately. Continue each morning (8:00 AM) until sign score is 0 or 1 for at least 24 hours.**

  * Liquid prednisolone: Prelone is 15 mg per 5 cc and Pediapred is 5 mg per 5 cc.
  ** If condition does not improve within two days after starting *oral steroid*, or if your child does not reach the *green zone* within seven days of treatment, see your doctor.

### Red Zone

**RED ZONE: Total asthma sign score 9 or more.**

**Follow this plan if sign score does not reach *Low Yellow Zone* within 10 minutes after taking inhaled *albuterol*, or drops back into *Red Zone* within four hours:**
- **Medicines to be taken:**
  - ✓ *Albuterol:* 0.__ cc by compressor-driven nebulizer.
  - ✓ *Oral steroid:* ____ mg.
- **Visit your doctor.**

The New Orleans intervention is distinctive in that it focuses on the practices of the primary care physicians who continue to improve their asthma care. All the equipment, materials, information, and referral services are designed to support the physician in providing effective asthma care, which will become an integral part of practice at all levels of PHCLa.

The asthma advocates, in turn, worked within their own practices to use and teach current concepts and techniques for asthma care to their colleagues. Through the conferences, physicians and nurses learned about and gained hands-on experience with peak flow meters and inhalation devices. During his visits to physicians' offices, the consultant discussed current asthma treatment and observed staff techniques for using equipment and educational materials.

Home health care staff are a significant unifying factor in the intervention. They ask physicians to prescribe home treatment plans based on the zones of the asthma diaries. They teach patients to assess the severity of asthma, how to use equipment, and how to follow their own progress. They report both to the primary care physicians and to the nurse case manager.

## Success Factors

The health services manager and the physician consultant agreed that each admission for asthma would be considered a failure of outpatient management by the physician or by the HMO unless proven otherwise. Providers are responsible for identifying problems that should be remedied to prevent a future admission. This is more productive than blaming the patient and avoids endless discussion of patient noncompliance.

This entire intervention is grounded in the experience of the health services manager, the nurse case manager, and the physician consultant. At least one of the three had experience in every major area of the program. The health services manager was experienced in initiating and implementing other programs that called for partnerships among physicians, vendors, and Principal staff. The nurse case manager had worked in utilization review and case management for several years. The consultant had guided or advised a dozen asthma interventions in practice settings and has assisted in creating asthma programs in schools, medical institutions, and Medicaid programs.

## Pitfall

The biggest concern the intervention faced was staff time. No one dropped other duties to participate, no staff were added, and the nurse case manager has been overextended. This is a problem that all similar interventions will face. The nurse case manager assigned to an intervention should be allotted an adequate amount of time to see each patient in the hospital, and sometimes the emergency room, and to coordinate their care thereafter.

### Adaptation

This intervention took place in an IPA model HMO. The general principles and concepts can be applied to any HMO or managed care practice, although it will be easier to implement in a staff model HMO, where patients and physicians are more concentrated and the manager's control is greater. This systems approach is also suitable for improving care of adults with asthma; PHCLa has recently expanded it to include the entire adult population at the plan. *One Minute Asthma*, the basic text for patients, is written at the sixth grade level and is available in Spanish.

### Projection

At the nine-month mark, most elements of the intervention are in place. PHCLa will soon begin analyzing inpatient care, emergency room care, physician prescribing habits, patient drug profiles, and patient satisfaction. Currently, some primary care physicians are taking full advantage of the resources offered. Within two years the majority of the physicians will be carrying out the entire program.

This systems approach to asthma care offers health plans a means for improving care and reducing unnecessary hospitalization. Most important, it provides health professionals with the knowledge, the tools, and the support they need to provide appropriate and current care for their asthma patients. It empowers the patients to play a significant role in improving the quality of their life.

## IMPROVING CARE FOR ADULTS WITH ASTHMA ACROSS THE CONTINUUM*

## Introduction

In the United States, the total prevalence of asthma has increased substantially, affecting 14.6 million individuals in 1994. Nationally, the overall costs for asthma in 1990 exceeded 6.2 billion dollars. Most patients have reversible symptoms that respond well to outpatient management. Annually, however, asthma accounts for nearly two million emergency department visits and more than 450,000 hospitalizations with an average length of stay of five days. The

*Source: Patti Ludwig-Beymer, RN, PhD, Sue Peterson, RN, BS, and Colleen Gorman, RN, MA, "Improving Care for Adults with Asthma across the Continuum," *Journal of Nursing Care Quality*, Vol. 12:6, Aspen Publishers, Inc., © August 1998.

number of physician office visits for asthma has also increased rapidly since 1990.

Based on data from the Centers for Disease Control and Prevention, prevalence rates of self-reported asthma increased 42 percent from 1982 through 1992, from 34.7 per 1,000 to 49.4 per 1,000. The overall death rate due to asthma increased 62 percent from 1982 through 1991, from 3,154 deaths to 5,106 deaths. A disproportionate increase has occurred in the African-American population. A study conducted in Chicago noted that between 1968 and 1991, asthma mortality did not significantly change for whites but increased 337 percent among African-Americans. Age-adjusted death rates for asthma are three times higher in black males than in white males and nearly three times higher in black females than in white females.

The need to improve care for patients with asthma has been well documented across the United States. Despite the publication of guidelines by the National Institutes of Health and many specialty groups, the delivery of care has not substantially changed. A group of health care providers with an integrated delivery system in Illinois wanted to affect a change in their care of asthma patients.

## Background

Before launching an adult asthma improvement team, the health care providers wanted to understand the needs of the primary service area communities surrounding eight system hospitals. Using zipcodes from the primary service areas surrounding each hospital, secondary data were analyzed. Because hospital admissions are regarded as an indication of poorly controlled asthma, the total number of hospitalizations at any Illinois hospital was obtained from the Illinois Hospital and HealthSystems Association. Healthy People 2000 set as a goal hospital admissions of 160 per 100,000. Hospital admissions were used for the numerator, and total population in the primary service area constituted the denominator. The total number of hospitalizations at any Illinois hospital for members of the communities is reported in Table 1. Tremendous variation exists within the eight hospital areas. The hospitals located within the city tend to have higher hospitalization rates for asthma; they also tend to have lower socioeconomic status, a greater proportion of African-Americans, and increased barriers to access to health care.

To identify care provided within the hospitals, the number of Emergency Department visits and hospitalizations were examined. ICD-9 (International Classification of Diseases-9th revision) codes were used for data analysis. In 1994, over 2,000 Emergency Department visits occurred for asthma in the survey hospital area. The same year, 900 adult patients were hospitalized with asthma as the principal diagnosis, and total charges for inpatient care exceeded 5.6 million dollars.

**Table 1.** Hospitalization for Asthma Reported in Primary Service Areas of Advocate Hospitals

| Hospital primary service area | Hospitalization rate* for all ages |
|---|---|
| Hospital A | 842 |
| Hospital B | 623 |
| Hospital C | 383 |
| Hospital D | 333 |
| Hospital E | 296 |
| Hospital F | 164 |
| Hospital G | 152 |
| Hospital H | 146 |

*Rates are per 100,000 population
Note: Numbers do not necessarily represent unique individuals.

In 1995, 832 hospitalizations and 2,111 Emergency Department visits occurred. In 1996, 857 adults were admitted for asthma and 2,310 were seen in the Emergency Department.

In addition, the practice patterns of physicians were surveyed prior to beginning the asthma initiative. Sixty physicians were asked to complete a mailed questionnaire, with 46 returning the questionnaire for a 76.7 percent return rate. Considerable variation was identified in their practice patterns. This variation included inpatient care (use and frequency of nebulized medications; use of steroids) and outpatient care (use of peak flow monitoring and classification of asthma).

Based on these findings, the health system believed that there were opportunities to improve patient care. The Adult Asthma Clinical Improvement Team was established to address these needs. The interdisciplinary team was composed of individuals from medicine (including specialists in allergy and immunology, emergency medicine, family practice, internal medicine, and pulmonology), nursing, pharmacy, respiratory care, and administration. Drawing heavily upon the national and international asthma guidelines, the team identified four major goals:

1. Improve management of adult asthma patients in outpatient settings, including physician prescribing practices.
2. Enhance partnership between patients and health care providers to improve patients' self-management skills and use of medical resources.
3. Improve identification and care of the most severe asthma patients.
4. Adopt and implement systemwide inpatient and emergency department care pathways.

## Outpatient Management

Related to improvements in the outpatient setting, a variety of clinical products was developed including Algorithms for Home Management of Acute Exacerbation of Asthma in Adults, Diagnosis of Asthma by Primary Care Physicians, and Exercise Induced Asthma; an Asthma Severity Classification; and an Environmental Assessment for Primary Care. Specialist referral criteria were developed to address the identification and referral of patients with the most severe asthma.

## Hospital Management

Emergency Department and inpatient care pathways were developed to further improve hospital-based care. These pathways standardized care for patients and included medical management as well as therapies and education.

## Patient Education

The team identified the need to establish a partnership between patients and health care providers. To accomplish this goal, patients needed to be empowered through education to take a more active role in their care. The team first identified components to be included in patient education materials and surveyed existing materials. Because no single educational piece met the needs identified, the team developed patient education materials using two formats: a patient education brochure and a wallet card. The patient education materials were designed to be used in multiple settings, including clinics, congregational health services, emergency departments, home health, hospitals, and physician offices.

The brochure provided general goals for controlling asthma. It then elaborated on three aspects of asthma management: an everyday treatment, medications, and how to handle an acute asthma episode. The brochure included checklists (lists of asthma triggers, early asthma symptoms) and write-in sections (personal best peak flow, medications). The document has a Flesch-Kincaid Reading level of less than sixth grade.

A wallet card was developed to summarize critical information contained in the brochure and make that information immediately accessible to patients. The trifold wallet card has a Flesch-Kincaid Reading Level grade of 4.3. The card includes information about medications and peak flows as well as a treatment plan for managing asthma symptoms.

## Communication

The work of the team was communicated throughout the system using a variety of techniques, including poster presentations, verbal presentations, and written communications. In particular, primary care physicians and pulmonologists were kept apprised of the project. The team also kept the Respiratory Council and Patient Care Council aware of their work.

## Implementation

The team identified three pilot sites to test both the products and the process of implementation. Implementation teams were formed at each site. These teams planned and delivered the site rollout, including communication, physician and staff education, and actual implementation of the protocol.

## Measurement Plan

The adult asthma team developed a measurement plan to evaluate the effectiveness of the program. The measurement plan included four primary areas: clinical outcomes, functional status, patient satisfaction, and resource utilization. When possible, the team used data that were retrievable from existing databases rather than creating additional data collection tools. For example, resource utilization was monitored using Transition Systems software whenever possible. Unfortunately, physician offices tended to be less automated than hospitals. To measure functional status, patient satisfaction, and the important process variables of medication use and peak flow meter access, a patient questionnaire was developed. A standard 20-item quality of life questionnaire with documented reliability and validity was identified for use in the patient questionnaire. Additional questions related to days missed from school or work, patient satisfaction, peak flow, and medications. The decision was reached to administer the questionnaire to adult patients with asthma when they were seen in the physician's office for any reason.

As part of the pilot evaluation, evaluation data were collected from patients, physicians, and other clinicians. In addition, patient functional status was measured. Physicians and other clinicians were very pleased with the protocol. A formal evaluation (see Table 2) revealed that physicians were most appreciative of the patient education materials. Other clinicians also found the patient education materials to be helpful.

Patients completed a quality of life survey at the time they were seen by the physician. As seen in Table 3, preliminary results reveal a population greatly affected by their disease. Patients will be asked to complete the survey 3 and 12 months after their initial treatment.

**Table 2.** Physician Office Feedback (n = 16)

| Asthma product | Number and % who have used the product | Number and % who found the product helpful (of those who used the product) | Number and % who found this to be the most helpful product |
|---|---|---|---|
| Patient education brochure | 13 (81%) | 11 (85%) | 6 (38%) |
| Wallet card | 11 (69%) | 7 (64%) | 5 (31%) |
| Asthma diagnosis algorithm | 10 (63%) | 7 (70%) | |
| Asthma classification scale | 13 (81%) | 10 (77%) | 1 (6%) |
| Environmental assessment | 9 (56%) | 8 (89%) | |
| Exercise-induced algorithm | 8 (50%) | 7 (88%) | |
| Chronic mild algorithm | 11 (69%) | 9 (82%) | |
| Medication algorithm | 10 (63%) | 8 (80%) | |
| Referral criteria | 5 (31%) | 4 (80%) | |
| Asthma flow sheet | 12 (75%) | 11 (92%) | 2 (13%) |
| Acute exacerbation algorithm | 10 (63%) | 9 (90%) | 1 (6%) |

Number and % physicians who report using guidelines has changed the way they care for patients
8 (50%)

Reported ways in which care has changed (Open-ended question)
- Use peak flows more often (×2)
- Take a more standardized approach
- Earlier use of home management and patient initiated PO steroids
- Spend more time teaching (×2)

## Lessons Learned

Talented clinicians, including physicians and other associates, were willing to participate in this clinical process improvement project without financial compensation. The team has learned a great deal together. Two major lessons occurred in the area of centralization versus decentralization and simultaneous implementation in hospitals and physician offices.

An early issue was the balance between centralization and decentralization. Each site needed to have autonomy to make the program work in its environment. For example, in some settings, respiratory care practitioners took the lead in providing education to physician office staff and patients. In other sites, registered nurses took ownership of this activity. In some emergency departments, the physician initiated the pathway. In others, the nurse initiated the pathway. In all situations, however, the need for collaboration in the delivery of care was emphasized.

However, some functions were better centralized. For example, pharmaceutical companies were anxious to partner with the health system in clinical improvement projects. Rather than negotiate with pharmaceutical companies at

**Table 3.** Asthma Quality of Life Questionnaire (AQLQ)*

| Scale | Sample (n = 36) | | | Asthma study (n = 71) |
|---|---|---|---|---|
| | Mean | Median | Standard deviation | Mean |
| Total AQLQ score | 32.2 | 39 | 19.2 | 28.1 |
| Breathlessness subscale | 9.1 | 8.5 | 4.3 | 8.7 |
| Mood disturbance subscale | 9.0 | 8.0 | 5.0 | 6.4 |
| Social disruption subscale | 8.4 | 5.0 | 8.6 | 4.5 |
| Concern for health subscale | 10.3 | 8.5 | 8.6 | 8.4 |

*Higher scores indicate that the patient perceives his/her quality of life negatively.

individual sites, this was handled centrally. Successful partnerships resulted in the funding of food for "learn at lunches," honorariums for physician educators, peak flow meters and placebo inhalers for training, and an unrestricted educational grant for the printing of materials and implementation of the measurement plan. In addition, ongoing support for the clinical improvement teams, including coaching, facilitation, database management, data analysis, and project management, was provided centrally.

Another important lesson learned from this project surrounds the challenges of implementing clinical improvements across the continuum. To truly improve care, clinical improvement activities must take place in all clinical settings, not only in hospitals. The hospitals within the system had a history of using continuous quality improvement techniques since 1990. This groundwork, along with the ability to communicate centrally, made effecting change within hospitals easy compared to implementing change in physician offices. Implementation in physician offices, on the other hand, required extensive resources. In addition, many primary care physician offices were not designed with space and personnel to provide in-depth education to patients with chronic diseases such as asthma. This is an issue that requires a long-term approach for resolution.

## Next Steps

Efforts to improve care for individuals with asthma continue throughout the system. Based on feedback from the pilot sites, the team is overseeing expansion of the pilot sites as well as implementation at the five remaining system hospitals and surrounding outpatient sites. Based on the team's data collection plan, data collection with feedback to the sites continues. Patient education materials are being translated into Spanish to meet the needs of that population. In addition, the team is currently revising the protocol to be in keeping with the 1997 asthma guidelines. Last, work on pediatric asthma is also needed to fulfill the system's mission.

## COSTS RELATED TO ASTHMA MANAGEMENT*

Costs of asthma include the direct expenses for hospital care, clinic visits, and medication, plus the indirect costs of time lost from school, work, or other duties. Direct costs may be easier to estimate than indirect costs, but asking a few

*Source: "Asthma Management and Prevention," NIH Publication No. 96-3659A, U.S. Department of Health and Human Services, National Institutes of Health, December 1995.

families how they are affected by asthma can give a good picture of the significance of all costs.

To estimate the direct costs of asthma in your community, start by estimating the costs for a day in the hospital and a visit to a rural clinic and by finding the actual cost of each medication used to treat asthma. Then collect data on the use of hospitals, rural clinics, and medications by patients with asthma. In a large community, it may be possible to collect data from a representative sample of hospitals and clinics and then generalize the sample to the entire community.

Remember that some hospital visits could be repeat visits by the same person with asthma. Thus for cost estimates, count the number of visits, not the number of patients. Once you have the number of visits and medications used by asthma patients, multiply these counts by the cost per visit and per medication to get the total estimated direct medical care costs related to asthma as illustrated in "Evaluating the Direct Costs of Asthma."

Despite limitations on available data, this type of cost evaluation can provide a lot of useful information in a short time and at low cost. A study of this kind was conducted in the South African Republic of Transkei in 1992, where it was found that 52 percent of direct medical care costs were for hospital-based care and were borne by 6 percent of the patients. The average hospital stay was 9 days—9 days of expensive care and 9 days of lost income. The study also found that Transkei's use of inhaled corticosteroids was limited by the high cost of that medicine.

Findings in Transkei raised the question of the value of allocating money for long-term preventive treatments in order to save hospitalization costs. When all costs were considered, it became clear that, for Transkei, the annual cost of providing inhaled corticosteroids was equivalent to the costs of 2.25 days in the hospital, or roughly one-fourth of the costs of a typical asthma-related hospitalization. Thus using long-term preventive treatment to manage asthma can be both less expensive and more beneficial.

Based on the estimates of the direct costs of asthma, your community can plan the best use of its asthma-related health care resources. Remember that taking public health measures such as dust mite control and education about asthma in addition to providing direct medical care may also lead to reductions in asthma-related expenses.

Indirect costs related to asthma have a significant impact. Untreated asthma can be very expensive. It may lead to frequent days of disability due to shortness of breath, wheezing, coughing, loss of sleep, or travel to a clinic or hospital. Children are unable to go to school, perform in all school activities, or help with family chores and thus contribute to the family's economic productivity. Adults lose productivity. Indirect costs may range from 50 to 100 percent of direct costs.

---

**Evaluating the Direct Costs of Asthma**

| | | | |
|---|---|---|---|
| (Cost 1 emergency care visit) | × (Emergency care visits for asthma) | = | Emergency costs |
| (Cost 1 day hospital care) | × (Days of hospital care for asthma) | = | Hospital care costs |
| (Cost 1 clinic visit) | × (Visits to clinic for asthma) | = | Clinic visit costs |
| (Cost 1 unit medication A) | × (Units of medication A for asthma) | = | Medication A costs |
| (Cost 1 unit medication B) | × (Units of medication B for asthma) | = | Medication B costs |
| (Cost 1 unit medication C) | × (Units of medication C for asthma) | = | Medication C costs |
| | ESTIMATED DIRECT COSTS | = | Sum of the above |

---

## PROGRAM DECISIONS*

Asthma management and prevention programs have many benefits. Individuals benefit from an improved quality of life. The community benefits from increased productivity in school and at work as well as from a smaller burden for treatment and special services. The economy benefits from reduced medical costs when medications are used to prevent attacks and expensive hospitalizations or emergency care.

To achieve these benefits, consider developing an asthma management and prevention program or adding asthma services to existing health programs. Any new asthma program must respond to the needs and resources of your community. Possible objectives for new programs include:

- Examining asthma care within the community to identify program needs and ways to improve the quality of care currently provided
- Increasing the use of peak flow measurements (especially in hospitals, clinics, and health centers), long-term preventive medications, environmental control of triggers, and written patient management plans among local health care providers
- Selecting medications for stepwise care appropriate for your area

- Assuring access to appropriate medications through community programs that involve insurers, hospitals, clinics, pharmacies, and other providers
- Identifying patients that carry the greatest risk of dying from asthma and those that consume the greatest resources and adopting specific programs in your clinic or hospital to serve these target patient groups
- Raising professional and public awareness of opportunities for asthma control with long-term management
- Screening high-risk population groups, such as young children or workers exposed to airborne chemicals, and providing asthma education and treatment referrals
- Initiating a communitywide prevention program for at-risk populations—for example, an antismoking campaign or a project that provides airtight mattress covers to pregnant women with asthma in their family
- Achieving consistent, high-quality asthma care and management throughout the community.

Program Development Questions and Resources offers information and questions for you to consider as actual program development decisions are made. The exhibit allows a sequence of steps: conducting a needs assessment, identifying objectives, developing a work plan, enlisting personnel resources, implementing the program, and evaluating and monitoring to assure continued success. At any stage of program planning, it may be helpful to review the questions and resource suggestions included in the exhibit. Of course, these suggested steps should be modified to meet your specific program needs.

---

*Source: "Asthma Management and Prevention," NIH Publication No. 96-3659A, U.S. Department of Health and Human Services, National Institutes of Health, December 1995.

**PROGRAM DEVELOPMENT QUESTIONS AND RESOURCES**

| Questions To Ask | Resources To Check |
|---|---|
| **CONDUCTING A NEEDS ASSESSMENT** | |
| What is the size of the local asthma problem?<br><br>What are the available asthma management and prevention services?<br><br>What treatments are currently used, available, affordable, and stable in your climate?<br><br>What areas have the greatest asthma problems?<br><br>Who are your neglected groups?<br><br>Where are interventions possible?<br><br>What are the public's perceptions of asthma?<br><br>With what institutions and groups can you collaborate? | Check hospital and clinic records for treatment of asthma-like symptoms.<br><br>Check school and work attendance records for evidence of asthma-related absences.<br><br>Interview representatives of relevant groups, health professionals, staff of existing services, and community leaders.<br><br>Interview individuals with asthma to identify barriers and areas of resistance.<br><br>Identify existing resources in institutions that can help with implementing the program (for example, supervision system, training unit, communications). |
| **IDENTIFYING OBJECTIVES** | |
| What do you want to achieve with this program?<br><br>Who do you want to reach?<br><br>How will you address public misperceptions?<br><br>Where will the program take place?<br><br>When will the program start and end?<br><br>How will you implement the program?<br><br>How will the project be financed? | Review materials and information gathered through the needs assessment.<br><br>Define specific objectives (for example, reduce hospitalizations, increase use of peak flow meters in clinics, increase the number of written plans, increase the number of patients discharged from the hospital with inhaled corticosteroids).<br><br>Define the priority target group.<br><br>Work with schools, workplaces, and other organizations offering asthma services to ensure compatibility and consistency.<br><br>Seek staff input in program development process.<br><br>Plan program to provide support, education, training, and coordination to overcome barriers. |
| **DEVELOPING A WORK PLAN** | |
| What tasks will need to be done to meet the objectives?<br><br>In what order should the tasks be done and by what date?<br><br>Where will the work take place?<br><br>Who will carry out, and supervise, the work?<br><br>How will the workers be trained?<br><br>What is the budget for the program?<br><br>Are adequate resources available?<br><br>Can additional funds be raised? | Meet with all interested in the program for recommendations and possible resource contributions.<br><br>Review other organizational plans for content and structure.<br><br>Consider estimating costs per unit of service and then calculate the number of units your resources will support.<br><br>Consider standardizing inhaler devices and medicines to reduce cost/storage/availability problems. |

*continues*

**Program Development Questions and Resources** continued

| Questions To Ask | Resources To Check |
|---|---|
| ENLISTING PERSONNEL RESOURCES | |
| Who will be responsible for this effort?<br><br>Who will be the resource persons for program activities, education, information, community support, and management problems?<br><br>How will you build in-house expertise?<br><br>How will training be encouraged?<br><br>Who will provide emergency care? | Current asthma management and prevention programs may have people with the skills and information needed.<br><br>Asthma specialists from any other areas may provide consultation.<br><br>Identify supervisors with technical and supportive skills in asthma management and prevention.<br><br>Enlist support from organizations working in other areas of health care. For example, ARI, TB, or primary care outreach programs may have answered similar questions and have a way to integrate asthma programs with their own. |
| IMPLEMENTING THE PROGRAM | |
| Who will announce the start of the program?<br><br>Who will provide support for supervisors and staff who are implementing the program?<br><br>Who will attend meetings to assess progress on a frequent and regular basis during early months of the program?<br><br>How will the program goals be monitored? | Identify current staff who support the program and have strong management skills to supervise the program.<br><br>Consider utilizing outside resources for training to introduce the program.<br><br>Prepare a plan to handle offers of assistance and support once the program is announced.<br><br>Integrate asthma education into program activities at every opportunity. |
| EVALUATING AND MONITORING TO ASSURE CONTINUED SUCCESS | |
| Are the objectives for the program being met?<br><br>Are regularly scheduled reviews being conducted?<br><br>Is the program moving forward in a timely manner?<br><br>Are the budget targets in line?<br><br>Is the quality of care consistently high?<br>  – Are patients on an appropriate step of therapy?<br>  – Are medication techniques demonstrated?<br>  – Are action plans given for stopping attacks?<br>  – Are written management plans given for long-term preventive medication and avoidance of triggers?<br><br>Are patients controlling their asthma?<br>  – Have patients participated in work or school and usual physical activities?<br>  – Have patients slept undisturbed?<br>  – Have patients required little or no quick-relief medication?<br>  – Have patients required little or no urgent care or medical treatment? | Use objectives and the work plan to develop a reporting and monitoring system.<br><br>Adjust the plan to respond to information gathered in evaluation.<br><br>Consider meetings with all staff regarding the success and problems with the program.<br><br>Develop a feedback mechanism to receive patient input. |
| SUCCESS | |

Source: "Asthma Management and Prevention," NIH Publication No. 96-3659A, U.S. Department of Health and Human Services, National Institutes of Health, December 1995.

# 2. Highlights of the National Asthma Education and Prevention Program's Expert Panel Report II: Guidelines for the Diagnosis and Management of Asthma

## PATHOGENESIS AND DEFINITION—KEY POINTS

- Asthma, whatever the severity, is a chronic inflammatory disorder of the airways. This has implications for the diagnosis, management, and potential prevention of the disease.
- The immunohistopathologic features of asthma include:
  - Denudation of airway epithelium
  - Collagen deposition beneath basement membrane
  - Edema
  - Mast cell activation
  - Inflammatory cell infiltration
    - Neutrophils (especially in sudden-onset, fatal asthma exacerbations)
  - Eosinophils
  - Lymphocytes (TH2-like cells)
- Airway inflammation contributes to airway hyperresponsiveness, airflow limitation, respiratory symptoms, and disease chronicity.
- Airway inflammation also contributes to several forms of airflow limitation, including acute bronchoconstriction, airway edema, mucus plug formation, and airway wall remodeling. These features lead to bronchial obstruction.
- Atopy, the genetic predisposition for the development of an IgE-mediated response to common aeroallergens, is the strongest identifiable predisposing factor for developing asthma.

Source: National Asthma Education and Prevention Program, *Expert Panel Report II: Guidelines for the Diagnosis and Management of Asthma*, National Heart, Lung, and Blood Institute, 1997.

# INITIAL ASSESSMENT AND DIAGNOSIS

## INITIAL ASSESSMENT AND DIAGNOSIS—KEY POINTS

- To establish a diagnosis of asthma, the clinician should determine that:
  - Episodic symptoms of airflow obstruction are present.
  - Airflow obstruction is at least partially reversible.
  - Alternative diagnoses are excluded.
- Recommended mechanisms to establish the diagnosis are:
  - Detailed medical history
  - Physical exam focusing on the upper respiratory tract, chest, and skin
  - Spirometry to demonstrate reversibility
- Additional studies may be considered to:
  - Evaluate alternative diagnoses
  - Identify precipitating factors
  - Assess severity
  - Investigate potential complications
- Recommendations are presented for referral for consultation or care to a specialist in asthma care.

Source: National Asthma Education and Prevention Program, *Expert Panel Report II: Guidelines for the Diagnosis and Management of Asthma*, National Heart, Lung, and Blood Institute, 1997.

## PERIODIC ASSESSMENT AND MONITORING—KEY POINTS

- The goals of therapy are to:
  - Prevent chronic and troublesome symptoms (e.g., coughing or breathlessness in the night, in the early morning, or after exertion)
  - Maintain (near) "normal" pulmonary function
  - Maintain normal activity levels (including exercise and other physical activity)
  - Prevent recurrent exacerbations of asthma and minimize the need for emergency department visits or hospitalizations
  - Provide optimal pharmacotherapy with least amount of adverse effects
  - Meet patients' and families' expectations of and satisfaction with asthma care
- Periodic assessments and ongoing monitoring of asthma are recommended to determine if the goals of therapy are being met. Measurements of the following are recommended:
  - Signs and symptoms of asthma
  - Pulmonary function
  - Quality of life/functional status
  - History of asthma exacerbations
  - Pharmacotherapy
  - Patient-provider communication and patient satisfaction
- Clinician assessment and patient self-assessment are the primary methods for monitoring asthma. Population-based assessment is beginning to be used by managed care organizations.
- Spirometry tests are recommended (1) at the time of initial assessment, (2) after treatment is initiated and symptoms and PEF have stabilized, and (3) at least every 1 to 2 years.
- Patients should be given a written action plan based on signs and symptoms and/or PEF; this is especially important for patients with moderate-to-severe persistent asthma or a history of severe exacerbations.
- Patients should be trained to recognize symptom patterns indicating inadequate asthma control and the need for additional therapy.
- Recommendations on how and when to do peak flow monitoring are presented.

Source: National Asthma Education and Prevention Program, *Expert Panel Report II: Guidelines for the Diagnosis and Management of Asthma*, National Heart, Lung, and Blood Institute, 1997.

## GENERAL GUIDELINES FOR REFERRAL TO AN ASTHMA SPECIALIST

**Based on the opinion of the Expert Panel, referral for consultation or care to a specialist in asthma care** (usually, a fellowship-trained allergist or pulmonologist; occasionally, other physicians with expertise in asthma management developed through additional training and experience) **is recommended when:**

- Patient has had a life-threatening asthma exacerbation.
- Patient is not meeting the goals of asthma therapy (see component 1—Periodic Assessment and Monitoring) after 3 to 6 months of treatment. An earlier referral or consultation is appropriate if the physician concludes that the patient is unresponsive to therapy.
- Signs and symptoms are atypical or there are problems in differential diagnosis.
- Other conditions complicate asthma or its diagnosis (e.g., sinusitis, nasal polyps, aspergillosis, severe rhinitis, vocal cord dysfunction, gastroesophageal reflux, chronic obstructive pulmonary disease).
- Additional diagnostic testing is indicated (e.g., allergy skin testing, rhinoscopy, complete pulmonary function studies, provocative challenge, bronchoscopy).
- Patient requires additional education and guidance on complications of therapy, problems with adherence, or allergen avoidance.

- Patient is being considered for immunotherapy.
- Patient has severe persistent asthma, requiring step 4 care (referral may be considered for patients requiring step 3 care; see component 3—Managing Asthma Long Term).
- Patient requires continuous oral corticosteroid therapy or high-dose inhaled corticosteroids or has required more than two bursts of oral corticosteroids in 1 year.
- Patient under age 3 and requires step 3 or 4 care (see component 3—Managing Asthma Long Term). When patient is under age 3 and requires step 2 care or initiation of daily long-term therapy, referral should be considered.
- Patient requires confirmation of a history that suggests that an occupational or environmental inhalant or ingested substance is provoking or contributing to asthma. Depending on the complexities of diagnosis, treatment, or the intervention required in the work environment, it may be appropriate in some cases for the specialist to manage the patient over a period of time or co-manage with the primary care provider.

In addition, patients with significant psychiatric, psychosocial, or family problems that interfere with their asthma therapy may need referral to an appropriate mental health professional for counseling or treatment. These characteristics have been shown to interfere with a patient's ability to adhere to treatment.

Source: National Asthma Education and Prevention Program, *Expert Panel Report II: Guidelines for the Diagnosis and Management of Asthma*, National Heart, Lung, and Blood Institute, 1997.

## KEY INDICATORS FOR CONSIDERING A DIAGNOSIS OF ASTHMA

Consider asthma and performing spirometry if *any* of these indicators are present.* These indicators are not diagnostic by themselves, but the presence of multiple key indicators increases the probability of a diagnosis of asthma. Spirometry is needed to establish a diagnosis of asthma.

- Wheezing—high-pitched whistling sounds when breathing out—especially in children. (Lack of wheezing and a normal chest examination do not exclude asthma.)
- History of any of the following:
  - Cough, worse particularly at night
  - Recurrent wheeze
  - Recurrent difficulty in breathing
  - Recurrent chest tightness
- Reversible airflow limitation and diurnal variation as measured by using a peak flow meter, for example:
  - Peak expiratory flow (PEF) varies 20 percent or more from PEF measurement on arising in the morning (before taking in inhaled short-acting beta$_2$-agonist) to PEF measurement in the early afternoon (after taking an inhaled short-acting beta$_2$-agonist).
- Symptoms occur or worsen in the presence of:
  - Exercise
  - Viral infection
  - Animals with fur or feathers
  - House-dust mites (in mattresses, pillows, upholstered furniture, carpets)
  - Mold
  - Smoke (tobacco, wood)
  - Pollen
  - Changes in weather
  - Strong emotional expression (laughing or crying hard)
  - Airborne chemicals or dusts
  - Menses
- Symptoms occur or worsen at night, awakening the patient.

*Eczema, hay fever, or a family history of asthma or atopic diseases are often associated with asthma, but they are not key indicators.

Source: National Asthma Education and Prevention Program, *Expert Panel Report II: Guidelines for the Diagnosis and Management of Asthma*, National Heart, Lung, and Blood Institute, 1997.

## IMPORTANCE OF SPIROMETRY IN ASTHMA DIAGNOSIS

Objective assessments of pulmonary function are necessary for the diagnosis of asthma because medical history and physical examination are not reliable means of excluding other diagnoses or of characterizing the status of lung impairment. Although physicians generally seem able to identify a lung abnormality as obstructive, they have a poor ability to assess the degree of airflow obstruction, or to predict whether the obstruction is reversible.

For diagnostic purposes, spirometry is generally recommended over measurements by a peak flow meter in the clinician's office because there is wide variability even in the best published peak expiratory flow reference values. Reference values need to be specific to each brand of peak flow meter, and such normative brand-specific values currently are not available for most brands. Peak flow meters are designed as monitoring, not as diagnostic, tools in the office. However, peak flow monitoring can establish peak flow variability and thus aid in the determination of asthma severity when patients have asthma symptoms and normal spirometry.

Source: National Asthma Education and Prevention Program, *Expert Panel Report II: Guidelines for the Diagnosis and Management of Asthma*, National Heart, Lung, and Blood Institute, 1997.

## SUGGESTED ITEMS FOR MEDICAL HISTORY

A detailed medical history of the new patient who is known or thought to have asthma should address the following items:

### 1. Symptoms

- Cough
- Wheezing
- Shortness of breath
- Chest tightness
- Sputum production

### 2. Pattern of Symptoms

- Perennial, seasonal, or both
- Continual, episodic, or both
- Onset, duration, frequency (number of days or nights, per week or month)
- Diurnal variations, especially nocturnal and on awakening in early morning

### 3. Precipitating and/or Aggravating Factors

- Viral respiratory infections
- Environmental allergens, indoor (e.g., mold, house-dust mite, cockroach, animal dander or secretory products) and outdoor (e.g., pollen)
- Exercise
- Occupational chemicals or allergens
- Environmental change (e.g., moving to a new home; going on vacation; and/or alterations in workplace, work processes, or materials used)
- Irritants (e.g., tobacco smoke, strong odors, air pollutants, occupational chemicals, dusts and particulates, vapors, gases, and aerosols)
- Emotional expressions (e.g., fear, anger, frustration, hard crying or laughing)
- Drugs (e.g., aspirin; beta-blockers, including eye drops; nonsteroidal anti-inflammatory drugs; others)
- Food, food additives, and preservatives (e.g., sulfites)
- Changes in weather, exposure to cold air
- Endocrine factors (e.g., menses, pregnancy, thyroid disease)

### 4. Development of Disease and Treatment

- Age of onset and diagnosis
- History of early-life injury to airways (e.g., bronchopulmonary dysplasia, pneumonia, parental smoking)
- Progress of disease (better or worse)
- Present management and response, including plans for managing exacerbations
- Need for oral corticosteroids and frequency of use
- Comorbid conditions

### 5. Family History

- History of asthma, allergy, sinusitis, rhinitis, or nasal polyps in close relatives

### 6. Social History

- Characteristics of home including age, location, cooling and heating system, wood-burning stove, humidifier, carpeting over concrete, presence of molds or mildew, characteristics of rooms where patient spends time (e.g., bedroom and living room with attention to bedding, floor covering, stuffed furniture)
- Smoking (patient and others in home or day care)
- Day care, workplace, and school characteristics that may interfere with adherence
- Social factors that interfere with adherence, such as substance abuse
- Social support/social networks
- Level of education completed
- Employment (if employed, characteristics of work environment)

### 7. Profile of Typical Exacerbation

- Usual prodromal signs and symptoms
- Usual patterns and management (what works?)

### 8. Impact of Asthma on Patient and Family

- Episodes of unscheduled care (emergency department, urgent care, hospitalization)
- Life-threatening exacerbations (e.g., intubation, intensive care unit admission)
- Number of days missed from school/work
- Limitation of activity, especially sports and strenuous work
- History of nocturnal awakening
- Effect on growth, development, behavior, school or work performance, and lifestyle
- Impact on family routines, activities, or dynamics
- Economic impact

### 9. Assessment of Patient's and Family's Perceptions of Disease

- Patient, parental, and spouse's or partner's knowledge of asthma and belief in the chronicity of asthma and in the efficacy of treatment
- Patient perception and beliefs regarding use and long-term effects of medications
- Ability of patient and parents, spouse, or partner to cope with disease
- Level of family support and patient's and parents', spouse's, or partner's capacity to recognize severity of an exacerbation
- Economic resources
- Sociocultural beliefs

This list does not represent a standardized assessment or diagnostic instrument. The validity and reliability of this list have not been assessed.

Source: National Asthma Education and Prevention Program, *Expert Panel Report II: Guidelines for the Diagnosis and Management of Asthma*, National Heart, Lung, and Blood Institute, 1997.

## SAMPLE QUESTIONS FOR THE DIAGNOSIS AND INITIAL ASSESSMENT OF ASTHMA

A "yes" answer to any question suggests that an asthma diagnosis is likely.

In the past 12 months

- Have you had a sudden severe episode or recurrent episodes of coughing, wheezing (high-pitched whistling sounds when breathing out), or shortness of breath?
- Have you had colds that "go to the chest" or take more than 10 days to get over?
- Have you had coughing, wheezing, or shortness of breath during a particular season or time of the year?
- Have you had coughing, wheezing, or shortness of breath in certain places or when exposed to certain things (e.g., animals, tobacco smoke, perfumes)?
- Have you used any medications that help you breathe better? How often?
- Are your symptoms relieved when the medications are used?

In the past 4 weeks, have you had coughing, wheezing, or shortness of breath:

- At night that has awakened you?
- In the early morning?
- After running, moderate exercise, or other physical activity?

These questions are examples and do not represent a standardized assessment or diagnostic instrument. The validity and reliability of these questions have not been assessed.

Source: National Asthma Education and Prevention Program, *Expert Panel Report II: Guidelines for the Diagnosis and Management of Asthma*, National Heart, Lung, and Blood Institute, 1997.

## DIAGNOSIS OF ASTHMA IN ADULTS AND CHILDREN

### DIAGNOSIS OF ASTHMA IN ADULTS AND CHILDREN OVER 5 YEARS OF AGE

Recurrent episodes of coughing or wheezing are almost always due to asthma in both children and adults. Cough can be the sole symptom.

Findings that increase the probability of asthma include:

**Medical history:**

- Episodic wheeze, chest tightness, shortness of breath, or cough.
- Symptoms worsen in presence of aeroallergens, irritants, or exercise.
- Symptoms occur or worsen at night, awakening the patient.
- Patient has allergic rhinitis or atopic dermatitis.
- Close relatives have asthma, allergy, sinusitis, or rhinitis.

**Physical examination of the upper respiratory tract, chest, and skin:**

- Hyperexpansion of the thorax
- Sounds of wheezing during normal breathing or a prolonged phase of forced exhalation
- Increased nasal secretions, mucosal swelling, sinusitis, rhinitis, or nasal polyps
- Atopic dermatitis/eczema or other signs of allergic skin problems

### DIAGNOSIS IN INFANTS AND CHILDREN YOUNGER THAN 5 YEARS OF AGE

Because children with asthma are often mislabeled as having bronchiolitis, bronchitis, or pneumonia, many do not receive adequate therapy.

- The diagnostic steps listed previously are the same for this age group except that spirometry is not possible. A trial of asthma medications may aid in the eventual diagnosis.
- **Diagnosis is not needed to *begin* to treat wheezing associated with an upper respiratory viral infection, which is the most common precipitant of wheezing in this age group.** Patients should be monitored carefully.

To establish an asthma diagnosis, determine the following:

1. **History or presence of episodic symptoms of airflow obstruction** (i.e., wheeze, shortness of breath, tightness in the chest, or cough). Asthma symptoms vary throughout the day; absence of symptoms at the time of the examination does not exclude the diagnosis of asthma.
2. **Airflow obstruction is at least partially reversible.** Use spirometry to:
   Establish airflow obstruction: $FEV_1$ <80 percent predicted; $FEV_1/FVC^*$ <65 percent or below the lower limit of normal. (If obstruction is absent, see Additional Tests for Adults and Children)
   Establish reversibility: $FEV_1$ increased $\geq$12 percent and at least 200 mL after using a short-acting inhaled beta$_2$-agonist (e.g., albuterol, terbutaline).
   **NOTE:** Older adults may need to take oral steroids for 2 to 3 weeks and then take the spirometry test to measure the degree of reversibility achieved. Chronic bronchitis and emphysema may coexist with asthma in adults. The degree of reversibility indicates the degree to which asthma therapy may be beneficial.
3. **Alternative diagnoses are excluded** (e.g., vocal cord dysfunction, vascular rings, foreign bodies, or other pulmonary diseases).

In general, $FEV_1$ predicted norms or reference values used for children should also be used for adolescents.

*$FEV_1$, forced expiratory volume in 1 second
FVC, forced vital capacity

- There are two general patterns of illness in infants and children who have wheezing with acute viral upper respiratory infections: a remission of symptoms in the preschool years and persistence of asthma throughout childhood. The factors associated with continuing asthma are allergies, a family history of asthma, and perinatal exposure to aeroallergens and passive smoke.

*continues*

**Diagnosis of Asthma** continued

### Additional Tests for Adults and Children

Additional tests may be needed when asthma is suspected but spirometry is normal, when coexisting conditions are suspected, or for other reasons.

These tests can aid diagnosis or confirm suspected contributors to asthma morbidity (e.g., allergens and irritants).

| Reasons for Additional Tests | The Tests |
| --- | --- |
| Patient has symptoms but spirometry is normal or near normal | Assess diurnal variation of peak flow over 1 to 2 weeks. <br><br> Refer to a specialist for bronchoprovocation with methacholine, histamine, or exercise; negative test may help rule out asthma. |
| Suspect infection, large airway lesions, heart disease, or obstruction by foreign object | Chest X-ray |
| Suspect coexisting chronic obstructive pulmonary disease, restrictive defect, or central airway obstruction | Additional pulmonary function studies <br> Diffusing capacity test |
| Suspect other factors contribute to asthma (These are not diagnostic tests for asthma.) | Allergy tests—skin or in vitro <br> Nasal examination <br> Gastroesophageal reflux assessment |

## PATIENT EDUCATION AFTER DIAGNOSIS

Identify the concerns the patient has about being diagnosed with asthma by asking: "What worries you most about having asthma?" What concerns do you have about your asthma?"

**Address the patient's concerns and make at least these key points:**

- **Asthma can be managed and the patient can live a normal life.**
- **Asthma can be controlled when the patient works together with the medical staff.** The patient plays a big role in monitoring asthma, taking medications, and avoiding things that can cause asthma episodes.
- **Asthma is a chronic lung disease characterized by inflammation of the airways.** There may be periods when there are no symptoms, but the airways are swollen and sensitive to some degree all of the time. Long-term anti-inflammatory medications are important to control airway inflammation.
- **Many things in the home, school, work, or elsewhere can cause asthma attacks** (e.g., secondhand tobacco smoke, allergens, irritants). An asthma attack (also called episodes, flareups, or exacerbations) occurs when airways narrow, making it harder to breathe.
- **Asthma requires long-term care and monitoring.** Asthma cannot be cured, but it can be controlled. Asthma can get better or worse over time and requires treatment changes.

Patient education should begin at the time of diagnosis and continue at every visit.

## ASSESSMENT OF ASTHMA SEVERITY

See "Classification of Asthma Severity" to estimate the severity of chronic asthma in patients of all age groups.

## GENERAL GUIDELINES FOR REFERRAL TO AN ASTHMA SPECIALIST

Based on the opinion of the Expert Panel, referral for consultation or care to a specialist in asthma care is recommended if assistance is needed for:

- **Diagnosis and assessment** (e.g., differential diagnosis is problematic, other conditions aggravate asthma, or confirmation is needed on the contribution of occupational or environmental exposures)
- **Specialized treatment and education** (e.g., considering patient for immunotherapy or providing additional education for allergen avoidance)
- **Other cases:**
  - Patient is not meeting the goals of asthma therapy after 3 to 6 months. An earlier referral or consultation is appropriate if the physician concludes that the patient is unresponsive to therapy.

*continues*

**Diagnosis of Asthma** continued

– Life-threatening asthma exacerbation occurred.

– Patient requires step 4 care or has used more than two bursts of oral steroids in 1 year. (Referral may be considered for patients requiring step 3 care.)

– Patient is younger than age 3 and requires step 3 or 4 care. Referral should be considered for patients under age 3 who require step 2 care.

An asthma specialist is usually a fellowship-trained allergist or pulmonologist or, occasionally, a physician with expertise in asthma management developed through additional training and experience.

**Patients with significant psychiatric, psychosocial, or family problems** that interfere with their asthma therapy should be referred to an appropriate mental health professional for counseling or treatment.

Source: "Practical Guide for the Diagnosis and Management of Asthma" (Based on the *Expert Panel Report II: Guidelines for the Diagnosis and Management of Asthma*), NIH Publication No. 97-4053, National Heart, Lung, and Blood Institute, National Institutes of Health, October 1997.

## CLASSIFICATION OF ASTHMA SEVERITY

**Clinical Features Before Treatment***

| | Symptoms** | Nighttime Symptoms | Lung Function |
|---|---|---|---|
| STEP 4<br>Severe Persistent | • Continual symptoms<br>• Limited physical activity<br>• Frequent exacerbations | Frequent | • $FEV_1$/PEF ≤60% predicted<br>• PEF variability >30% |
| STEP 3<br>Moderate<br>Persistent | • Daily symptoms<br>• Daily use of inhaled short-acting beta$_2$-agonist<br>• Exacerbations affect activity<br>• Exacerbations ≥2 times a week; may last days | >1 time a week | • $FEV_1$/PEF >60%–<80% predicted<br>• PEF variability >30% |
| STEP 2<br>Mild Persistent | • Symptoms >2 times a week but <1 time a day<br>• Exacerbations may affect activity | >2 times a month | • $FEV_1$/PEF ≥80% predicted<br>• PEF variability 20–30% |
| STEP 1<br>Mild Intermittent | • Symptoms ≤2 times a week<br>• Asymptomatic and normal PEF between exacerbations<br>• Exacerbations brief (from a few hours to a few days); intensity may vary | ≤2 times a month | • $FEV_1$/PEF ≥80% predicted<br>• PEF variability <20% |

*The presence of one of the features of severity is sufficient to place a patient in that category. An individual should be assigned to the most severe grade in which any feature occurs. The characteristics noted in this figure are general and may overlap because asthma is highly variable. Furthermore, an individual's classification may change over time.

**Patients at any level of severity can have mild, moderate, or severe exacerbations. Some patients with intermittent asthma experience severe and life-threatening exacerbations separated by long periods of normal lung function and no symptoms.

Source: National Asthma Education and Prevention Program, *Expert Panel Report II: Guidelines for the Diagnosis and Management of Asthma*, National Heart, Lung, and Blood Institute, 1997.

## DIFFERENTIAL DIAGNOSTIC POSSIBILITIES FOR ASTHMA

**INFANTS AND CHILDREN**

**Upper Airway Diseases**

- Allergic rhinitis and sinusitis

**Obstruction Involving Large Airways**

- Foreign body in trachea or bronchus
- Vocal cord dysfunction
- Vascular rings or laryngeal webs
- Laryngotracheomalacia, tracheal stenosis, or bronchostenosis
- Enlarged lymph nodes or tumor

**Obstructions Involving Small Airways**

- Viral bronchiolitis or obliterative bronchiolitis
- Cystic fibrosis
- Bronchopulmonary dysplasia
- Heart disease

**Other Causes**

- Recurrent cough not due to asthma
- Aspiration from swallowing mechanism dysfunction or gastroesophageal reflux

**ADULTS**

- Chronic obstructive pulmonary disease (chronic bronchitis or emphysema)
- Congestive heart failure
- Pulmonary embolism
- Laryngeal dysfunction
- Mechanical obstruction of the airways (benign and malignant tumors)
- Pulmonary infiltration with eosinophilia
- Cough secondary to drugs (angiotensin-converting enzyme [ACE] inhibitors)
- Vocal cord dysfunction

Source: National Asthma Education and Prevention Program, *Expert Panel Report II: Guidelines for the Diagnosis and Management of Asthma*, National Heart, Lung, and Blood Institute, 1997.

## PERIODIC ASSESSMENT AND MONITORING*

### Goals of Therapy

The purpose of periodic assessment and ongoing monitoring is to determine whether the goals of asthma therapy are being achieved. The goals of therapy are as follows:

- Prevent chronic and troublesome symptoms (e.g., coughing or breathlessness in the night, in the early morning, or after exertion)
- Maintain (near) "normal" pulmonary function
- Maintain normal activity levels (including exercise and other physical activity)
- Prevent recurrent exacerbations of asthma and minimize the need for emergency department visits or hospitalizations
- Provide optimal pharmacotherapy with minimal or no adverse effects
- Meet patients' and families' expectations of and satisfaction with asthma care

---

*Source: National Asthma Education and Prevention Program, *Expert Panel Report II: Guidelines for the Diagnosis and Management of Asthma*, National Heart, Lung, and Blood Institute, 1997.

### Assessment Measures

**The Expert Panel recommends ongoing monitoring in the six areas listed below to determine whether the goals of therapy are being met.** The assessment measures for monitoring these six areas are described in this section and are **recommended based on the opinion of the Expert Panel**.

- Monitoring signs and symptoms of asthma
- Monitoring pulmonary function
  - Spirometry
  - Peak flow monitoring
- Monitoring quality of life/functional status
- Monitoring history of asthma exacerbations
- Monitoring pharmacotherapy
- Monitoring patient-provider communication and patient satisfaction

### *Monitoring Signs and Symptoms of Asthma*

**Every patient with asthma should be taught to recognize symptom patterns that indicate inadequate asthma control.** Symptom monitoring should be used as a means to determine the need for intervention, including additional medication, in the context of an action plan.

**Symptoms and clinical signs of asthma should be assessed at each health care visit through physical examination and appropriate questions.** This is crucial to optimal asthma care.

Detailed patient recall of symptoms decreased over time; therefore, **the Expert Panel recommends that any detailed symptoms history be based on a short (2 to 4 weeks) recall period.** For example, the clinician may choose to assess over a 2-week, 3-week, or 4-week recall period (see exhibit titled "Components of the Clinician's Follow-Up Assessment: Sample Routine Clinical Assessment Questions"). Symptom assessment for periods longer than 4 weeks should reflect more global symptom assessment, such as inquiring whether the patient's asthma has been better or worse since the last visit and inquiring whether the patient has encountered any particular difficulties during specific seasons or events. The exhibit provides an example of a set of questions that can be used to characterize both global (long-term recall) and recent (short-term recall) asthma symptoms.

In addition, **any assessment of the patient's symptom history should include at least three key symptom expressions**:

- Daytime asthma symptoms (including wheezing, cough, chest tightness, or shortness of breath)
- Nocturnal awakening as a result of asthma symptoms
- Asthma symptoms early in the morning that are not improved 15 minutes after inhaling a short-acting beta$_2$-agonist

## Monitoring Pulmonary Function

In addition to assessing symptoms, it is also important to periodically assess pulmonary function. The main methods are spirometry and peak flow monitoring.

Regular monitoring of pulmonary function is particularly important for asthma patients who do not perceive their symptoms until airflow obstruction is severe. Currently, there is no readily available method of detecting the "poor perceivers." The literature reports that patients who had a near-fatal asthma exacerbation, as well as older patients, are more likely to have poor perception of airflow obstruction.

**Spirometry. The Expert Panel recommends that spirometry tests be done (1) at the time of initial assessment; (2) after treatment is initiated and symptoms and peak expiratory flow (PEF) have stabilized, to document attainment or (near) "normal" airway function; and (3) at least every 1 to 2 years to assess the maintenance of airway function.**

Spirometry may be indicated more often than every one to two years, depending on the clinical severity and response to

management. Spirometry with measurement of the FEV$_1$ is also useful:

- As a periodic (e.g., yearly) check on the accuracy of the peak flow meter
- When more precision is desired in measuring lung function (e.g., when evaluating response to bronchodilator or nonspecific airway responsiveness or when assessing response to a "step down" in pharmacotherapy)
- When PEF results are unreliable (e.g., in some very young or elderly patients or when neuromuscular or orthopedic problems are present) and the physician needs the quality checks that are available only with spirometry.

For routine monitoring at most outpatient visits, measurement of PEF with a peak flow meter is generally a sufficient assessment of pulmonary function, particularly in mild intermittent, mild persistent, and moderate persistent asthma.

**Peak Flow Monitoring.** Peak expiratory flow provides a simple, quantitative, and reproducible measure of the existence and severity of airflow obstruction. PEF can be measured with inexpensive and portable peak flow meters. *It must be stressed that peak flow meters are designed as tools for ongoing* monitoring, *not* diagnosis. Because the measurement of PEF is dependent on effort and technique, patients need instructions, demonstrations, and frequent reviews of technique.

Peak flow monitoring can be used for short-term monitoring, managing exacerbations, and daily long-term monitoring. When used in these ways, the patient's measured personal best is the most appropriate reference value. Four studies have found that comprehensive asthma self-management programs, in which peak flow monitoring was a component, achieved significant improvements in health outcomes. Thus far, the few studies that have isolated a comparison of peak flow and symptom monitoring have not been sufficient to assess the relative contributions of each to asthma management. The literature does suggest which patients may benefit most from peak flow monitoring. The Expert Panel concludes, on the basis of this literature and the Panel's opinion, that:

- Patients with moderate-to-severe persistent asthma should learn how to monitor their PEF and have a peak flow meter at home.
- Peak flow monitoring during exacerbations of asthma is recommended for patients with moderate-to-severe persistent asthma to:
  - Determine severity of the exacerbation

## COMPONENTS OF THE CLINICIAN'S FOLLOW-UP ASSESSMENT: SAMPLE ROUTINE CLINICAL ASSESSMENT QUESTIONS

### MONITORING SIGNS AND SYMPTOMS

**Global Assessment**

- "Has your asthma been better or worse since your last visit?"

**Recent Assessment**

- "In the past 2 weeks, how many days have you:
  - Had problem with coughing, wheezing, shortness of breath, or chest tightness during the day?"
  - Awakened at night from sleep because of coughing or other asthma symptoms?"
  - Awakened in the morning with asthma symptoms that did not improve within 15 minutes of inhaling a short-acting beta$_2$-agonist?"
  - Had symptoms while exercising or playing?"

### MONITORING PULMONARY FUNCTION

**Lung Function**

- "What is the highest and lowest your peak flow has been since your last visit?"
- "Has your peak flow dropped below ___L/min (80 percent of personal best) since your last visit?"
- "What did you do when this occurred?"

**Peak Flow Monitoring Technique**

- "Please show me how you measure your peak flow."
- "When do you usually measure your peak flow?"

### MONITORING QUALITY OF LIFE/FUNCTIONAL STATUS

- "Since your last visit, how many days has your asthma caused you to:
  - Miss work or school?"
  - Reduce your activities?"
  - (For caregivers) Change your activity because of your child's asthma?"
- "Since your last visit, have you had any unscheduled or emergency department visits or hospital stays?"

### MONITORING EXACERBATION HISTORY

- "Since your last visit, have you had any episodes/times when your asthma symptoms were a lot worse than usual?"
  - If yes—"What do you think caused the symptoms to get worse?"
  - If yes—"What did you do to control the symptoms?

- "Have there been any changes in your home or work environment (e.g., new smokers or pets)?"

### MONITORING PHARMACOTHERAPY

**Medications**

- "What medications are you taking?"
- "How often do you take each medication?" "How much do you take each time?"
- "Have you missed or stopped taking any regular doses of your medications for any reason?"
- "Have you had trouble filling your prescriptions (e.g., for financial reasons, not on formulary)?"
- "How many puffs of your short-acting inhaled beta$_2$-agonist (quick-relief medicine) do you use per day?"
- "How many _____ [name of short-acting inhaled beta$_2$-agonist] inhalers [or pumps] have you been through in the past month?
- "Have you tried any other medicines or remedies?

**Side Effects**

- "Has your asthma medicine caused you any problems?"
  - shakiness, nervousness, bad taste, sore throat, cough, upset stomach

**Inhaler Technique**

"Please show me how you use your inhaler."

### MONITORING PATIENT-PROVIDER COMMUNICATION AND PATIENT SATISFACTION

- "What questions have you had about your asthma daily self-management plan and action plan?"
- "What problems have you had following your daily self-management plan? Your action plan?"
- "Has anything prevented you from getting the treatment you need for your asthma from me or anyone else?"
- "Have the costs of your asthma treatment interfered with your ability to get asthma care?"
- "How satisfied are you with your asthma care?"
- "How can we improve your asthma care?"
- "Let's review some important information:"
  - "When should you increase your medications? Which medication(s)?"
  - "When should you call me [your doctor or nurse practitioner]? Do you know the after-hours phone number?"
  - "If you can't reach me, what emergency department would you go to?"

Note: These questions are examples and do not represent a standardized assessment instrument. The validity and reliability of these questions have not been assessed.

Source: National Asthma Education and Prevention Program, *Expert Panel Report II: Guidelines for the Diagnosis and Management of Asthma*, National Heart, Lung, and Blood Institute, 1997.

–Guide therapeutic decisions in the home, clinician's office, or emergency department

- Long-term daily peak flow monitoring is helpful in managing patients with moderate-to-severe persistent asthma to:

–Detect early changes in disease status that require treatment

–Evaluate responses to changes in therapy

–Provide assessment of severity for patients with poor perception of airflow obstruction

–Afford a quantitative measure of impairment

- If long-term daily peak flow monitoring is not used, a short-term (2 to 3 weeks) period of peak flow monitoring is recommended to:

–Evaluate responses to changes in chronic maintenance therapy

–Identify temporal relationship between changes in PEF and exposure to environmental or occupational irritants or allergens. It may be necessary to record PEF four or more times a day.

–Identify the individual patient's personal best PEF

- The Expert Panel does not recommend long-term daily peak flow monitoring for patients with mild intermittent or mild persistent asthma unless the patient/family and/ or clinician find it useful in guiding therapeutic decisions. Any patient who develops severe exacerbations may benefit from peak flow monitoring.

Limitations of long-term peak flow monitoring include:

- Difficulty in maintaining adherence to monitoring, often due to inconvenience, lack of required level of motivation, or lack of a specific treatment plan based on PEF
- Potential for incorrect readings related to poor technique, misinterpretation, or device failure

Whether peak flow monitoring, symptom monitoring, or a combination of approaches is used, the Expert Panel believes that self-monitoring is important to the effective self-management of asthma. The nature and intensity of self-monitoring should be individualized, based on such factors as asthma severity, patient's ability to perceive airflow obstruction, availability of peak flow meters, and patient preferences.

**It is the opinion of the Expert Panel that, regardless of the type of monitoring used, patients should be given a written action plan and be instructed to use it. The Panel believes it is especially important to give a written action plan to patients with moderate-to-severe persistent asthma and any patient with a history of severe exacerbations.** The action plan will describe the actions patients should take based on their signs and symptoms and/or PEF. The clinician should periodically review the plan, revise it as necessary,

and confirm that the patient knows what to do if his or her asthma gets worse.

## Monitoring Quality of Life/Functional Status

To determine whether the goals of asthma therapy are being met, it is crucial to examine how the disease expression and control are affecting the patient's quality of life. Several dimensions of quality of life may be important to track, including physical function, role function, and mental health function. Several comprehensive survey instruments, such as the SF-36, have been developed for general use for patient populations. In addition, a number of asthma-specific quality-of-life survey instruments have been developed, several of which appear promising. However, certain concerns preclude the Expert Panel from recommending the general adoption of these instruments at this time, such as the lack of experience with the use of the instruments in clinical practice and the time involved in administering the surveys. **The Expert Panel does recommend that at least several key areas of quality of life be periodically assessed for each person with asthma.** These include:

- Any missed work or school due to asthma
- Any reduction in usual activities (either home/work/ school or recreation/exercise)
- Any disturbances in sleep due to asthma
- Any change in caregiver activities due to a child's asthma (for caregivers of children with asthma)

The exhibit titled "Components of the Clinician's Follow-Up Assessment" provides a set of questions that the Expert Panel recommends for use in characterizing quality-of-life concerns for persons with asthma.

## Monitoring History of Asthma Exacerbations

Exacerbations of asthma are characterized by periods of increased symptoms and reduced lung function, which may result in diminished ability to perform usual activities. Exacerbations may be brought on by exposures to irritants or sensitizers in the home, work, or general environment. Infections, certain medications, and a number of other medical conditions, as well as insufficient or ineffective therapy, also may trigger exacerbations.

**During periodic assessments, clinicians should question the patient and evaluate any records of patient self-monitoring to detect exacerbations, both self-treated and those treated by other health care providers.** It is important to evaluate the frequency, severity, and causes of exacerbations. The patient should be asked about precipitating exposures and other factors. Specific inquiry into unscheduled visits to providers, telephone calls for assistance, and

## RECOMMENDATIONS ON HOW TO MONITOR PEAK FLOW

**The Expert Panel recommends that patients who are using a peak flow meter be instructed on how to establish their personal best peak expiratory flow and use it as the basis of their action plan.** Meters used to measure PEF should meet American Thoracic Society recommendations for monitoring devices.

The patient's personal best PEF can be estimated after a 2- to 3-week period in which the patient records PEF two to four times per day. The personal best value is usually achieved in the early afternoon measurement after maximal therapy has stabilized the patient. A course of oral corticosteroids may be needed to establish the personal best PEF. The patient's personal best value should be reassessed periodically to account for progression of disease in children and adults and for growth in children. Occasionally, a PEF value is recorded that is markedly higher than other values. This may be due to "spitting" (especially if the peak flow meter mouthpiece is small) or coughing into the peak flow meter, as well as other reasons that are not well understood. Therefore, caution should be used in establishing a personal best value when an outlying value is observed. Children with moderate-to-severe asthma should repeat the short-term monitoring period every 6 months to establish changes in personal best PEF that occur with growth.

**Patients requiring daily peak flow monitoring should measure their PEF on waking from sleep in the morning before taking a bronchodilator,** if the patient uses a bronchodilator. When the morning PEF is below 80 percent of the patient's personal best, PEF should be measured more than once a day (again, before taking a bronchodilator). This recommendation is based not on scientific data, but on the logic of reducing delays in treatment. The additional measurements of PEF during the day will enable patients to detect if their asthma is continuing to worsen or is improving after taking medication. If their asthma is worsening, they will have the opportunity to quickly respond to this. In addition, periodically having patients take their PEF first thing in the morning and in the early afternoon for 1 to 2 weeks will assess airflow variability, which is an indicator of the current level of the patient's asthma severity.

**It is the Expert Panel's opinion that, in general, PEF below 80 percent of the patient's personal best before bronchodilator inhalation indicates a need for additional medication. PEF below 50 percent indicates a severe asthma exacerbation.** These cutpoints of 80 and 50 percent of the personal best are somewhat arbitrary. The emphasis is not on a specific PEF value but, rather, on a patient's change from personal best or from one reading to the next. Cutpoints should be tailored to individual patients' needs and PEF patterns.

Cutpoints may be easier to use and remember when they are adapted to a traffic light system. In this system, for example, the green zone (80 to 100 percent of personal best) signals good control, the yellow zone (50 to less than 80 percent of personal best) signals caution, and the red zone (below 50 percent of personal best) signals a medical alert. Because the yellow zone includes a wide spectrum of asthma severity, clinicians may consider recommending different interventions for a high yellow zone (e.g., 65 to less than 80 percent of personal best) and a low yellow zone (e.g., 50 to less than 65 percent of personal best).

**The Expert Panel recommends that patients use the same peak flow meter over time** and bring their peak flow meter for use at every followup visit. Using the same brand of meter is recommended because different brands of meters can give significantly different values and because lung function varies across racial and ethnic populations. Thus, there is no universal normative standard for PEF. In addition, brand-specific normative values are not available for most peak flow meters.

Despite this variability across different brands of peak flow meters, measurements from the same meter and meters of the same brand are fairly consistent in measuring PEF. Thus, once patients establish their personal best PEF on their own meter, they can obtain reliable and clinically meaningful readings of their PEF. However, at each visit, the patient's peak flow meter should be inspected. At least once a year, or any time there is a question about the validity of peak flow meter readings, PEF values from the portable peak flow meter and from laboratory spirometry should be compared.

When patients replace their peak flow meter, it is prudent to have them reestablish their personal best PEF with the new meter, regardless of whether the replacement meter is the same brand as the original. Action plan cutpoints also may need to be modified. The durability and consistency over time of peak flow meters have not been adequately studied to provide guidance on when a peak flow meter needs to be replaced.

Source: National Asthma Education and Prevention Program, *Expert Panel Report II: Guidelines for the Diagnosis and Management of Asthma*, National Heart, Lung, and Blood Institute, 1997.

use of urgent or emergency care facilities may be helpful. Severity can be estimated by the increased need for oral corticosteroids. Control of asthma can be assessed by the increased need for short-acting beta$_2$-agonist. Finally, any hospitalizations should be documented, including the facility, duration of stay, and any use of critical care or intubation. The clinician then can request summaries of all care received to facilitate continuity of care.

## Monitoring Pharmacotherapy

To ensure the effectiveness of pharmacotherapy, it is essential that the drug regimen be based on a sound rationale and that it be monitored on an ongoing basis. **Based on the opinion of the Expert Panel, the following factors should be monitored: patient adherence to the regimen, inhaler technique, level of usage of as-needed inhaled short-acting beta$_2$-agonist, frequency of oral corticosteroid "burst" therapy, changes in dosage of inhaled anti-inflammatory or other long-term-control medications, and side effects of medications.** It is also crucial that the clinician determine that the patient is on the appropriate step of pharmacotherapy and has an up-to-date, written daily self-management plan and action plan.

## Monitoring Patient-Provider Communication and Patient Satisfaction

**Health care providers should routinely assess the effectiveness of patient/provider communication** (see the exhibit titled "Components of the Clinician's Follow-Up Assessment"). Open and unrestricted communication among the clinician, the patient, and the family is essential to ensure successful self-management by the patient with asthma. Every effort should be made to encourage open discussion of concerns and expectation of therapy.

Patient satisfaction with their asthma care and resolution of fears and concerns are important goals and will increase adherence to the treatment plan. **Two aspects of patient satisfaction should be monitored: satisfaction with asthma control and satisfaction with the quality of care.**

## Assessment Methods

Each of the key measures used in the periodic assessment of asthma (i.e., signs and symptoms, pulmonary function, quality of life, history of exacerbations, pharmacotherapy, and patient-provider communication and patient satisfaction) can be obtained by several methods. The principal methods include clinician assessment and patient (and/or parent or caregiver) self-assessment. In addition, population-based assessment of asthma care is being developed in the managed care field.

## Clinician Assessment

Clinical assessment of asthma should be obtained via medical history and physical examination with appropriate pulmonary function testing. Optimal history assessment may be best achieved via a consistent set of questions (see the exhibit titled "Components of the Clinician's Follow-Up

Assessment). **Patients with mild intermittent or mild persistent asthma that has been under control for at least 3 months should be seen by a clinician about every 6 months.** This is a rough guideline based on the opinion of the Expert Panel. The exact frequency of clinician visits is a matter of clinical judgment. **Patients with uncontrolled and/or severe persistent asthma and those needing additional supervision to help them follow their treatment plan need to be seen more often.**

## Patient Self-Assessment

Self-assessment by the patient and/or family is important to determine from *their* perspective whether the asthma is well controlled. Two methods are recommended: a daily diary and a periodic self-assessment form to be filled out by the patient and/or family member at the time of the followup visits to the clinician (see the form titled "Sample Patient Self-Assessment Sheet for Follow-Up Visits").

- The daily diary should include the key factors to be monitored at home: symptoms and/or peak flow, medication use, and restricted activity.
- The periodic self-assessment sheet completed at office visits is intended to capture the patient's and family's impression of asthma control, self-management skills, and overall satisfaction with care.

Patients are less likely to see completion of diaries and forms as a burden if they receive feedback from the clinician that allows them to see value in self-monitoring. Monitoring with a daily diary will be most useful to patients whose asthma is not yet under control and who are trying new treatments. It is also useful for those who need help identifying environmental or occupational exposures that make their asthma worse.

## Population-Based Assessment

Asthma care is of increasing interest in various health care settings. Important regulatory organizations for the industry (e.g., the National Committee on Quality Assurance) have included the care of persons with asthma as a key indicator of quality of managed care. In this context, periodic population-based assessment of asthma care has begun to emerge as an issue for patients and their clinical providers. This type of assessment often uses population experience, such as hospitalization or emergency department visit rates, to examine care within different clinical settings and among different providers. Complex standardized population surveys (including lengthy health status instruments) are being tested experimentally in the managed care setting.

# Sample Patient Self-Assessment Sheet for Follow-Up Visits

Name: _____   Date: _____

How many days in the past week have you had chest tightness, cough, shortness of breath, or wheezing (whistling in your chest)?    ___0  ___1  ___2  ___3  ___4  ___5  ___6  ___7

How many nights in the past week have you had chest tightness, cough, shortness of breath, or wheezing (whistling in your chest)?    ___0  ___1  ___2  ___3  ___4  ___5  ___6  ___7

Do you perform peak flow readings at home?    ___ yes   ___ no

If yes, did you bring your peak flow chart?    ___ yes   ___ no

How many days in the past week has asthma restricted your physical activity?    ___0  ___1  ___2  ___3  ___4  ___5  ___6  ___7

Have you had any asthma attacks since your last visit?    ___ yes   ___ no

Have you had any unscheduled visits to a doctor, including to the emergency department, since your last visit?    ___ yes   ___ no

How many puffs of your short-acting inhaled beta$_2$-agonist (quick-relief medicine) do you use per day?    _____
Average number of puffs per day

How many of your short-acting inhaled beta$_2$-agonist inhalers did you go through over the past month?    _____
Number of inhalers in past month

What questions or concerns would you like to discuss with the doctor?

_____

_____

How well controlled is your asthma in your opinion?    ___ very well controlled
___ somewhat controlled
___ not well controlled

How satisfied are you with your asthma care?    ___ very satisfied
___ somewhat satisfied
___ not satisfied

Note: These questions are examples and do not represent a standardized assessment instrument. The validity and reliability of these questions have not been assessed.

Source: National Asthma Education and Prevention Program, *Expert Panel Report II: Guidelines for the Diagnosis and Management of Asthma*, National Heart, Lung, and Blood Institute, 1997.

# CONTROL OF FACTORS CONTRIBUTING TO ASTHMA SEVERITY

## CONTROL OF FACTORS CONTRIBUTING TO ASTHMA SEVERITY—KEY POINTS

- Exposure of asthma patients to irritants or allergens to which they are sensitive has been shown to increase asthma symptoms and precipitate asthma exacerbations.
- For at least those patients with persistent asthma on daily medications, the clinician should:
  - Identify allergen exposures
  - Use the patient's history to assess sensitivity to seasonal allergens
  - Use skin testing or in vitro testing to assess sensitivity to perennial indoor allergens
  - Assess the significance of positive tests in context of patients' medical history
- Patients with asthma at any level of severity should avoid:
  - Exposure to allergens to which they are sensitive.
  - Exposure to environmental tobacco smoke.
  - Exertion when levels of air pollution are high.
  - Use of beta-blockers.
  - Sulfite-containing and other foods to which they are sensitive.
  - Aspirin and nonsteroidal anti-inflammatory drugs if they have a history of sensitivity; if they have severe persistent asthma, they should be counseled regarding the potential risk attendant with use of these drugs.
- Patients should be treated for rhinitis, sinusitis, and gastroesophageal reflux, if present.
- Patients with persistent asthma should be given an annual influenza vaccine.

Source: National Asthma Education and Prevention Program, *Expert Panel Report II: Guidelines for the Diagnosis and Management of Asthma*, National Heart, Lung, and Blood Institute, 1997.

# Assessment Questions for Environmental and Other Factors That Can Make Asthma Worse

## INHALANT ALLERGENS

Does the patient have symptoms year round? (If yes, ask the following questions. If no, see next set of questions.)

____ Does the patient keep pets indoors? What type? _____

____ Does the patient have moisture or dampness in any room of his or her home (e.g., basement)? (Suggests house-dust mites, molds.)

____ Does the patient have mold visible in any part of his or her home? (Suggests molds.)

____ Has the patient seen cockroaches in his or her home in the past month? (Suggests significant cockroach exposure.)

____ Assume exposure to house-dust mites unless patient lives in a semiarid region. However, if a patient living in a semiarid region uses a swamp cooler, exposure to house-dust mites must still be assumed.

Do symptoms get worse at certain times of the year? (If yes, ask when symptoms occur.)

____ Early spring? (trees)

____ Late spring? (grasses)

____ Late summer to autumn? (weeds)

____ Summer and fall? (*Alternaria, Cladosporium*)

## TOBACCO SMOKE

____ Does the patient smoke?

____ Does anyone smoke at home or work?

____ Does anyone smoke at the child's day care?

## INDOOR/OUTDOOR POLLUTANTS AND IRRITANTS

____ Is a wood-burning stove or fireplace used in the patient's home?

____ Are there unvented stoves or heaters in the patient's home?

____ Does the patient have contact with other smells or fumes from perfumes, cleaning agents, or sprays?

## WORKPLACE EXPOSURES

____ Does the patient cough or wheeze during the week, but not on weekends when away from work?

____ Do the patient's eyes and nasal passages get irritated soon after arriving at work?

*continues*

**Assessment Questions** continued

\_\_\_\_ Do coworkers have similar symptoms?

\_\_\_\_ What substances are used in the patient's work site? (Assess for sensitizers.)

## RHINITIS

\_\_\_\_ Does the patient have constant or seasonal nasal congestion and/or postnasal drip?

## GASTROESOPHAGEAL REFLUX

\_\_\_\_ Does the patient have heartburn?

\_\_\_\_ Does food sometimes come up into the patient's throat?

\_\_\_\_ Has the patient had coughing, wheezing, or shortness of breath at night in the past 4 weeks?

\_\_\_\_ Does the infant vomit followed by cough or have wheezing cough at night? Are symptoms worse after feeding?

## SULFITE SENSITIVITY

\_\_\_\_ Does the patient have wheezing, coughing, or shortness of breath after eating shrimp, dried fruit, or processed potatoes, or after drinking beer or wine?

## MEDICATION SENSITIVITIES AND CONTRAINDICATIONS

\_\_\_\_ What medications does the patient use now (prescription and nonprescription)?

\_\_\_\_ Does the patient use eyedrops? What type?

\_\_\_\_ Does the patient use any medications that contain beta-blockers?

\_\_\_\_ Does the patient ever take aspirin or other nonsteroidal anti-inflammatory drugs?

\_\_\_\_ Has the patient ever had symptoms of asthma after taking any of these medications?

Note: These questions are examples and do not represent a standardized assessment or diagnostic instrument. The validity and reliability of these questions have not been assessed.

Source: National Asthma Education and Prevention Program, *Expert Panel Report II: Guidelines for the Diagnosis and Management of Asthma*, National Heart, Lung, and Blood Institute, 1997.

## COMPARISON OF SKIN TESTS WITH IN VITRO TESTS

**Advantages of Skin Tests**

- Less expensive than in vitro tests
- Results are available within 1 hour
- More sensitive than in vitro tests
- Results are visible to the patient. This may encourage compliance with environmental control measures.

**Advantages of RAST and Other In Vitro Tests**

- Do not require knowledge of skin testing technique
- Do not require availability of allergen extracts
- Can be performed on patients who are taking medications that suppress the immediate skin test (antihistamines, antidepressants)
- No risk of systemic reactions
- Can be done for patients with extensive eczema

Source: National Asthma Education and Prevention Program, *Expert Panel Report II: Guidelines for the Diagnosis and Management of Asthma*, National Heart, Lung, and Blood Institute, 1997.

# Patient Interview Questions for Assessing the Clinical Significance of Positive Allergy Tests

- **Animal Dander.** If there are pets in the patient's home and the patient is sensitive to dander of that species of animal, the likelihood that animal dander allergy is contributing to asthma symptoms is increased if answers to the following questions are affirmative. However, absence of positive responses does not exclude a contribution of animal dander to the patient's symptoms.

  _____ Do nasal, eye, or chest symptoms appear in a room where carpets are being or have just been vacuumed?

  _____ Do nasal, eye, or chest symptoms improve when away from home for a week or longer?

  _____ Do the symptoms become worse the first 24 hours after returning home?

- **House-Dust Mites.** Mite allergy is more likely to be a contributing factor to asthma severity if answers to the following questions are affirmative. However, absence of a positive response does not exclude a contribution of mite allergen to the patient's symptoms.

  _____ Do nasal, eye, or chest symptoms appear in a room where carpets are being or have just been vacuumed?

  _____ Does making a bed cause nasal, eye, or chest symptoms?

- **Outdoor Allergens (Pollens and Outdoor Molds).** Contribution of pollens and outdoor molds in causing asthma symptoms is suggested by a positive answer to this question:

  _____ Is asthma consistently worse in spring, summer, fall, or parts of the growing season?

  Usually, if pollen or mold spores are causing increased asthma symptoms, the patient will also have symptoms of allergic rhinitis—sneezing, itching nose and eyes, runny and obstructed nose.

- **Indoor Fungi (Molds).** Contribution of indoor molds in causing asthma symptoms is suggested by a positive answer to this question:

  _____ Do nasal, eye, or chest symptoms appear in damp or moldy rooms, such as basements?

These questions are provided as examples for the clinician. The validity and reliability of these questions have not been assessed.

Source: National Asthma Education and Prevention Program, *Expert Panel Report II: Guidelines for the Diagnosis and Management of Asthma*, National Heart, Lung, and Blood Institute, 1997.

## SUMMARY OF CONTROL MEASURES FOR ENVIRONMENTAL FACTORS THAT CAN MAKE ASTHMA WORSE

### ALLERGENS

Reduce or eliminate exposure to the allergen(s) the patient is sensitive to, including:

- **Animal dander:** Remove animal from house or, at a minimum, keep animal out of patient's bedroom and seal or cover with a filter air ducts that lead to bedroom.
- **House-dust mites:**
  - *Essential:* Encase mattress in an allergen-impermeable cover; encase pillow in an allergen-impermeable cover or wash it weekly; wash sheets and blankets on the patient's bed in hot water weekly (water temperature of $\geq 130°F$ is necessary for killing mites).
  - *Desirable:* Reduce indoor humidity to less than 50 percent; remove carpets from the bedroom; avoid sleeping or lying on upholstered furniture; remove carpets that are laid on concrete.
- **Cockroaches:** Use poison bait or traps to control. Do not leave food or garbage exposed.
- **Pollens (from trees, grass, or weeds) and outdoor molds:** To avoid exposures, adults should stay indoors with windows closed during the season in which they have problems with outdoor allergens, especially during the afternoon.
- **Indoor mold:** Fix all leaks and eliminate water sources associated with mold growth; clean moldy surfaces. Consider reducing indoor humidity to less than 50 percent.

### TOBACCO SMOKE

Advise patients and others in the home who smoke to stop smoking or to smoke outside the home. Discuss ways to reduce exposure to other sources of tobacco smoke, such as from day care providers and the workplace.

### INDOOR/OUTDOOR POLLUTANTS AND IRRITANTS

Discuss ways to reduce exposures to the following:

- Wood-burning stoves or fireplaces
- Unvented stoves or heaters
- Other irritants (e.g., perfumes, cleaning agents, sprays)

Source: National Asthma Education and Prevention Program, *Expert Panel Report II: Guidelines for the Diagnosis and Management of Asthma*, National Heart, Lung, and Blood Institute, 1997.

## EVALUATION AND MANAGEMENT OF WORK-AGGRAVATED ASTHMA AND OCCUPATIONAL ASTHMA

### EVALUATION

**Potential for Workplace-Related Symptoms**

- Recognized sensitizers (e.g., isocyanates, plant or animal products)
- Irritants* or physical stimuli (e.g., cold/heat, dust, humidity)
- Coworkers may have similar symptoms

**Patterns of Symptoms (in relation to work exposures)**

- Improvement during vacations or days off (make take a week or more)
- Symptoms may be immediate (<1 hour), delayed (most commonly, 2 to 8 hours after exposure), or nocturnal
- Initial symptoms may occur after high-level exposure (e.g., spill)

**Documentation of Work-Relatedness of Airflow Limitation**

- Serial charting for 2 to 3 weeks (2 weeks at work and up to 1 week off work as needed to identify or exclude work-related changes in peak expiratory flow)
  - Record when symptoms and exposures occur
  - Record when a bronchodilator is used
  - Measure and record peak flow every 2 hours while awake
- Immunologic tests
- Referral for further confirmatory evaluation (e.g., bronchial challenges)

### MANAGEMENT

**Work-Aggravated Asthma**

- Work with on-site health care providers or managers/supervisors
- Discuss avoidance, ventilation, respiratory protection, tobacco smoke-free environment

**Occupationally Induced Asthma**

- Recommend complete cessation of exposure to initiating agent

*Material Safety Data Sheets may be helpful for identifying respiratory irritants, but many sensitizers are not listed.

Source: National Asthma Education and Prevention Program, *Expert Panel Report II: Guidelines for the Diagnosis and Management of Asthma*, National Heart, Lung, and Blood Institute, 1997.

# PHARMACOLOGIC THERAPY

## MEDICATIONS—KEY POINTS

### LONG-TERM CONTROL MEDICATIONS

- **Corticosteroids.** Most potent and effective anti-inflammatory medication currently available. Inhaled form is used in the long-term control of asthma. Systemic corticosteroids are often used to gain prompt control of the disease when initiating long-term therapy.
- **Cromolyn sodium and nedocromil.** Mild-to-moderate anti-inflammatory medications. May be used as initial choice for long-term-control therapy for children. Can also be used as preventive treatment prior to exercise or unavoidable exposure to known allergens.
- **Long-acting beta$_2$-agonists.** Long-acting bronchodilator used concomitantly with anti-inflammatory medications for long-term control of symptoms, especially nocturnal symptoms. Also prevents exercise-induced bronchospasm (EIB).
- **Methylxanthines.** Sustained-release theophylline is a mild-to-moderate bronchodilator used principally as adjuvant to inhaled corticosteroids for prevention of nocturnal asthma symptoms. May have mild anti-inflammatory effect.

- **Leukotriene modifiers.** Zafirlukast, a leukotriene receptor antagonist, or zileuton, a 5-lipoxygenase inhibitor, may be considered an alternative therapy to low doses of inhaled corticosteroids or cromolyn or nedocromil for patients $\geq 12$ years of age with mild persistent asthma, although further clinical experience and study are needed to establish their roles in asthma therapy.

### QUICK-RELIEF MEDICATIONS

- **Short-acting beta$_2$-agonists.** Therapy of choice for relief of acute symptoms and prevention of EIB.
- **Anticholinergics.** Ipratropium bromide may provide some additive benefit to inhaled beta$_2$-agonists in severe exacerbations. May be an alternative bronchodilator for patients who do not tolerate inhaled beta$_2$-agonists.
- **Systemic corticosteroids.** Used for moderate-to-severe exacerbations to speed recovery and prevent recurrence of exacerbations.

Source: National Asthma Education and Prevention Program, *Expert Panel Report II: Guidelines for the Diagnosis and Management of Asthma*, National Heart, Lung, and Blood Institute, 1997.

## SPECIAL ISSUES REGARDING SAFETY—KEY POINTS

### SHORT-ACTING INHALED BETA$_2$-AGONISTS

- Short-acting beta$_2$-agonists are the most effective medication for relieving acute bronchospasm.
- Increasing use of short-acting beta$_2$-agonists or the use of more than one canister in 1 month indicates inadequate control of asthma and the need for initiating or intensifying anti-inflammatory therapy.
- Regularly scheduled, daily use of short-acting beta$_2$-agonists is generally not recommended.

### LONG-ACTING INHALED BETA$_2$-AGONISTS

- Long-acting beta$_2$-agonists (salmeterol) can be beneficial to patients when added to inhaled corticosteroid therapy, especially to control nighttime symptoms. Daily use of long-acting beta$_2$-agonists should generally not exceed 84 mcg (salmeterol; four puffs).
- *Salmeterol is not to be used for treatment of acute symptoms or exacerbations.*
- Patient education regarding correct use of salmeterol is critical.
- Patients should be instructed not to stop anti-inflammatory therapy while taking salmeterol even though their symptoms may significantly improve.

### INHALED CORTICOSTEROIDS

- Inhaled corticosteroids are the most effective long-term therapy available for mild, moderate, or severe persistent asthma; in general, inhaled corticosteroids are well tolerated and safe at the recommended dosages.
- The potential but small risk of adverse events from the use of inhaled corticosteroids is well balanced by their efficacy.
- To reduce the potential for adverse effects, the following measures are recommended:
  - Administer inhaled corticosteroids with spacers/holding chambers.
  - Advise patients to rinse their mouths (rinse and spit) following inhalation.
  - Use the lowest possible dose of inhaled corticosteroid to maintain control.
  - To maintain control of asthma (especially for nocturnal symptoms), consider adding a long-acting inhaled beta$_2$-agonist to a low-to-medium dose of inhaled corticosteroid rather than using a higher dose of inhaled corticosteroid.
  - For children, monitor growth.
  - For postmenopausal women, consider supplements of calcium (1,000 to 1,500 mg per day) and vitamin D (400 units a day). Estrogen replacement therapy, where appropriate, may be considered for patients on doses that exceed 1,000 mcg of inhaled corticosteroid a day.

### INHALED CORTICOSTEROIDS AND LINEAR GROWTH IN CHILDREN

- The potential risks of inhaled corticosteroids are well balanced by their benefits.
- Growth rates are highly variable in children. Short-term evaluations may not be predictive of attaining final adult height.
- Poorly controlled asthma may delay growth in children.
- In general, children with asthma tend to have longer periods of reduced growth rates prior to puberty (males > females).
- The potential for adverse effects on linear growth from inhaled corticosteroids appears to be dose dependent. In treating children with *mild-to-moderate persistent asthma*, medium-dose inhaled corticosteroid therapy may be associated with a possible, but not predictable, adverse effect on linear growth. The clinical significance of this potential systemic effect has yet to be determined. High doses of inhaled corticosteroids have greater potential for growth suppression.
- Use of high doses of inhaled corticosteroids with children with severe persistent asthma has significantly less potential for having an adverse effect on linear growth than oral systemic corticosteroids.
- A majority of studies of the use of inhaled corticosteroids by children have not demonstrated an effect on growth, but a few have identified growth delay. Some caution (e.g., monitoring growth, stepping down therapy when possible) is suggested while this issue is studied further.

Source: National Asthma Education and Prevention Program, *Expert Panel Report II: Guidelines for the Diagnosis and Management of Asthma*, National Heart, Lung, and Blood Institute, 1997.

## LONG-TERM CONTROL MEDICATIONS

| Name/Products | Indications/Mechanisms | Potential Adverse Effects | Therapeutic Issues |
|---|---|---|---|
| **Corticosteroids (Glucocorticoids)** | | | |
| *Inhaled*<br>Beclomethasone dipropionate<br>Budesonide<br>Flunisolide<br>Fluticasone propionate<br>Triamcinolone acetonide | *Indications*<br>• Long-term prevention of symptoms; suppression, control and reversal of inflammation.<br>• Reduce need for oral corticosteroid.<br><br>*Mechanisms*<br>• **Anti-inflammatory.** Block late reaction to allergen and reduce airway hyperresponsiveness. Inhibit cytokine production, adhesion protein activation, and inflammatory cell migration and activation.<br>• Reverse beta$_2$-receptor down-regulation. Inhibit microvascular leakage. | • Cough, dysphonia, oral thrush (candidiasis).<br>• In high doses, systemic effects may occur, although studies are not conclusive, and clinical significance of these effects has not been established (e.g., adrenal suppression, osteoporosis, growth suppression, and skin thinning and easy bruising). | • Spacer/holding chamber devices and mouth washing after inhalation decrease local side effects and systemic absorption.<br>• Preparations are not absolutely interchangeable on a mcg or per puff basis. New delivery devices may provide greater delivery to airways, which may affect dose.<br>• The risks of uncontrolled asthma should be weighed against the limited risks of inhaled corticosteroids. The potential but small risk of adverse events is well balanced by their efficacy.<br>• Dexamethasone is not included because it is highly absorbed and has long-term suppressive side effects. |
| *Systemic*<br>Methylprednisolone<br>Prednisolone<br>Prednisone | *Indications*<br>• For short-term (3-10 days) "burst": to gain prompt control of inadequately controlled persistent asthma.<br>• For long-term prevention of symptoms in severe persistent asthma: suppression, control, and reversal of inflammation.<br><br>*Mechanisms*<br>• Same as inhaled. | • Short-term use: reversible abnormalities in glucose metabolism, increased appetite, fluid retention, weight gain, mood alteration, hypertension, peptic ulcer, and rarely aseptic necrosis of femur.<br>• Long-term use: adrenal axis suppression, growth suppression, dermal thinning, hypertension, diabetes, Cushing's syndrome, cataracts, muscle weakness, and—in rare instances—impaired immune function.<br>• Consideration should be given to coexisting condition that could be worsened by systemic corticosteroids, such as herpes virus infections, *Varicella*, tuberculosis, hypertension, peptic ulcer, and *Strongyloides*. | Use at lowest effective dose. For long-term use, alternate-day a.m. dosing produces least toxicity. If daily doses are required, one study shows improved efficacy with no increase in adrenal suppression when administered at 3 p.m. rather than in the morning. |

*continues*

**Long-Term Control Medications** continued

| Names/Products | Indications/Mechanisms | Potential Adverse Effects | Therapeutic Issues |
|---|---|---|---|
| **Cromolyn Sodium and Nedocromil**<br><br>Cromolyn<br>Nedocromil | *Indications*<br><br>• Long-term prevention of symptoms; may modify inflammation.<br><br>• Preventive treatment prior to exposure to exercise or known allergen.<br><br>*Mechanisms*<br><br>• **Anti-inflammatory.** Block early and late reaction to allergen. Interfere with chloride channel function. Stabilize mast cell membranes and inhibit activation and release of mediators from eosinophils and epithelial cells.<br><br>• Inhibit acute response to exercise, cold dry air, and $SO_2$. | 15 to 20 percent of patients complain of an unpleasant taste from nedocromil. | • Therapeutic response to cromolyn and nedocromil often occurs within 2 weeks, but a 4- to 6-week trial may be needed to determine maximum benefit.<br><br>• Dose of cromolyn MDI (1 mg/puff) may be inadequate to affect airway hyper-responsiveness. Nebulizer delivery (20 mg/ampule) may be preferred for some patients.<br><br>• Safety is the primary advantage of these agents. |
| **Long-Acting Beta$_2$-Agonists**<br><br>*Inhaled*<br>Salmeterol | *Indications*<br><br>• Long-term prevention of symptoms, especially nocturnal symptoms, *added to anti-inflammatory therapy.*<br><br>• Prevention of exercise-induced bronchospasm.<br><br>• *Not to be used to treat acute symptoms or exacerbations.*<br><br>*Mechanisms*<br><br>• **Bronchodilation.** Smooth muscle relaxation following adenylate cyclase activation and increase in cyclic AMP producing functional antagonism of bronchoconstriction.<br><br>• In vitro, inhibit mast cell mediator release, decrease vascular permeability, and increase mucociliary clearance.<br><br>• Compared to short-acting inhaled beta$_2$-agonist, salmeterol (but not formoterol) has slower onset of action (15 to 30 minutes) but longer duration (>12 hours). | • Tachycardia, skeletal muscle tremor, hypokalemia, prolongation of QT$_c$ interval in overdose.<br><br>• A diminished bronchoprotective effect may occur within 1 week of chronic therapy. Clinical significance has not been established. | • *Not to be used to treat acute symptoms or exacerbations.*<br><br>• Clinical significance of potentially developing tolerance is uncertain because studies show symptom control and bronchodilation are maintained.<br><br>• Should not be used in place of anti-inflammatory therapy.<br><br>• May provide more effective symptom control when added to standard doses of inhaled corticosteroid compared to increasing the corticosteroid dosage. |
| *Oral*<br>Albuterol, sustained-release | | | • *Inhaled long-acting beta$_2$-agonists are preferred because they are longer acting and have fewer side effects than oral sustained-release agents.* |

continues

**Long-Term Control Medications** continued

| Names/Products | Indications/Mechanisms | Potential Adverse Effects | Therapeutic Issues |
|---|---|---|---|
| **Methylxanthines**<br><br>Theophylline, sustained-release tablets and capsules | *Indications*<br>• Long-term control and prevention of symptoms, especially nocturnal symptoms.<br><br>*Mechanisms*<br>• **Bronchodilation.** Smooth muscle relaxation from phosphodiesterase inhibition and possibly adenosine antagonism.<br><br>• May affect eosinophilic infiltration into bronchial mucosa as well as decrease T-lymphocyte numbers in epithelium.<br><br>• Increases diaphragm contractility and mucociliary clearance. | • Dose-related acute toxicities include tachycardia, nausea and vomiting, tachyarrhythmias (SVT), central nervous system stimulation, headache, seizures, hematemesis, hyperglycemia, and hypokalemia.<br><br>• Adverse effects at usual therapeutic doses include insomnia, gastric upset, aggravation of ulcer or reflux, increase in hyperactivity in some children, difficulty in urination in elderly males with prostatism. | • Maintain steady-state serum concentrations between 5 and 15 mcg/mL. Routine serum concentration monitoring is essential due to significant toxicities, narrow therapeutic range, and individual differences in metabolic clearance. Absorption and metabolism may be affected by numerous factors, which can produce significant changes in steady-state serum theophylline concentrations.<br><br>• Not generally recommended for exacerbations. There is minimal evidence for added benefit to optimal doses of inhaled beta$_2$-agonists. Serum concentration monitoring is mandatory. |
| **Leukotriene Modifiers**<br><br>Zafirlukast tablets | *Indications*<br>• Long-term control and prevention of symptoms in mild persistent asthma for patients ≥12 years of age.<br><br>*Mechanisms*<br>• **Leukotriene receptor antagonist:** selective competitive inhibitor of LTD4 and LTE4 receptors. | • No specific adverse effects to date. As with any new drug, there is possibility of rare hypersensitivity or idiosyncratic reactions that cannot usually be detected in initial premarketing trials. One reported case of reversible hepatitis and hyperbilirubinemia; high concentrations may develop in patients with liver impairment. | • Administration with meals decreases bioavailability; take at least 1 hour before or 2 hours after meals.<br><br>• Inhibits the metabolism of warfarin and increases prothrombin time; it is a competitive inhibitor of the CYP2C9 hepatic microsomal isozymes. (It has not affected elimination of terfenadine, theophylline, or ethinyl estradiol drugs metabolized by the CYP3A4 isozymes.) |
| Zileuton tablets | *Indications*<br>• Long-term control and prevention of symptoms in mild persistent asthma for patients ≥12 years of age.<br><br>*Mechanisms*<br>• **5-lipoxygenase inhibitor.** | • Elevation of liver enzymes has been reported. Limited case reports of reversible hepatitis and hyperbilirubinemia. | • Zileuton is microsomal CYP3A4 enzyme inhibitors that can inhibit the metabolism of terfenadine, warfarin, and theophylline. Doses of these drugs should be monitored accordingly.<br><br>• Monitor hepatic enzymes (ALT). |

Source: National Asthma Education and Prevention Program, *Expert Panel Report II: Guidelines for the Diagnosis and Management of Asthma*, National Heart, Lung, and Blood Institute, 1997.

## INHALED STEROIDS: THE MOST EFFECTIVE LONG-TERM-CONTROL MEDICATION FOR ASTHMA

**The daily use of inhaled steroids results in the following:**

- Asthma symptoms will diminish. Improvement will continue gradually (see Table A).

- Occurrence of severe exacerbations is greatly reduced.

- Use of quick-relief medication decreases (see Table B).

- Lung function improves significantly, as measured by peak flow, $FEV_1$, and airway hyperresponsiveness.

Problems due to asthma may return if patients stop taking inhaled steroids.

**Frequency of dosing**

Once-daily dosing with inhaled steroids for patients with mild asthma and twice-a-day dosing for many other patients, even with high doses of some preparations, have been effective.

### Table A

Daily Inhaled Steroids Control Moderate Persistent Asthma in Children 7 to 16 Years Old: Reduced Symptomatic Days*

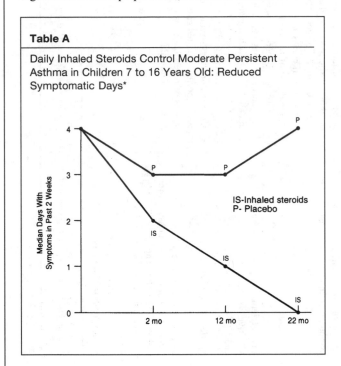

### Table B

Inhaled Steroids Control Asthma in Adults: Significant Reduction in Need for Quick-Relief Medicine*

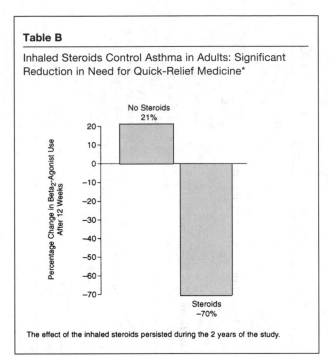

The effect of the inhaled steroids persisted during the 2 years of the study.

**\*Other endpoints**—$FEV_1$, peak flow, airway hyperresponsiveness, and symptoms—significantly improved relative to the placebo group over 22 months of the children's study (N=116) and over 2 years in the adult study (N=103).

Source: "Practical Guide for the Diagnosis and Management of Asthma" (Based on the *Expert Panel Report II: Guidelines for the Diagnosis and Management of Asthma*), NIH Publication No. 97-4053, National Heart, Lung, and Blood Institute, National Institutes of Health, October 1997.

## QUICK-RELIEF MEDICATIONS

| Name/Products | Indications/Mechanisms | Potential Adverse Effects | Therapeutic Issues |
|---|---|---|---|
| **Short-Acting Inhaled Beta$_2$-Agonists**<br><br>Albuterol<br>Bitolterol<br>Pirbuterol<br>Terbutaline | *Indications*<br><br>• Relief of acute symptoms; quick-relief medication.<br><br>• Preventive treatment prior to exercise for exercise-induced bronchospasm.<br><br>*Mechanisms*<br><br>• **Bronchodilation.** Smooth muscle relaxation following adenylate cyclase activation and increase in cyclic AMP producing functional antagonism of bronchoconstriction. | Tachycardia, skeletal muscle tremor, hypokalemia, increased lactic acid, headache, hyperglycemia. Inhaled route, in general, causes few systemic adverse effects. Patients with preexisting cardiovascular disease, especially the elderly, may have adverse cardiovascular reactions with inhaled therapy. | • Drugs of choice for acute bronchospasm. Inhaled route has faster onset, fewer adverse effects, and is more effective than systemic routes. The less beta$_2$-selective agents (isoproterenol, metaproterenol, isoetharine, and epinephrine) are not recommended due to excessive cardiac stimulation. Albuterol liquid is not recommended.<br><br>• For patients with mild intermittent asthma, regularly scheduled daily use neither harms nor benefits asthma control. Regularly scheduled daily use is not generally recommended.<br><br>• Increasing use or lack of expected effect indicates inadequate asthma control. >1 canister a month (e.g., albuterol-200 puffs per canister) may indicate overreliance on this drug; ≥2 canisters in 1 month poses additional adverse risks.<br><br>• For patients frequently using beta$_2$-agonist, anti-inflammatory medication should be initiated or intensified. |
| **Anticholinergics**<br><br>Ipratropium bromide | *Indications*<br><br>• Relief of acute bronchospasm (see Therapeutic Issues column).<br><br>*Mechanisms*<br><br>• **Bronchodilation.** Competitive inhibition of muscarinic cholinergic receptors.<br><br>• Reduces intrinsic vagal tone to the airways. May block reflex bronchoconstriction secondary to irritants or to reflux esophagitis.<br><br>• May decrease mucus gland secretion. | Drying of mouth and respiratory secretions, increased wheezing in some individuals, blurred vision if sprayed in eyes. | • Reverses only cholinergically mediated bronchospasm; does not modify reaction to antigen. Does not block exercise-induced bronchospasm.<br><br>• May provide additive effects to beta$_2$-agonist but has slower onset of action.<br><br>• Is an alternative for patients with intolerance to beta$_2$-agonists.<br><br>• Treatment of choice for bronchospasm due to beta-blocker medication. |

*continues*

**Quick-Relief Medications** continued

| Name/Products | Indications/Mechanisms | Potential Adverse Effects | Therapeutic Issues |
|---|---|---|---|
| **Corticosteroids**<br><br>*Systemic:*<br>Methylprednisolone<br>Prednisolone<br>Prednisone | *Indications*<br><br>• For moderate-to-severe exacerbations to prevent progression of exacerbation, reverse inflammation, speed recovery, and reduce rate of relapse.<br><br>*Mechanisms*<br><br>• **Anti-inflammatory.** | • Short-term use: reversible abnormalities in glucose metabolism, increased appetite, fluid retention, weight gain, mood alteration, hypertension, peptic ulcer, and rarely aseptic necrosis of femur.<br><br>• Consideration should be given to coexisting conditions that could be worsened by systemic corticosteroids, such as herpes virus infections, *Varicella*, tuberculosis, hypertension, peptic ulcer, and *Strongyloides*. | • Short-term therapy should continue until patient achieves 80% PEF personal best or symptoms resolve. This usually requires 3 to 10 days but may require longer.<br><br>• There is no evidence that tapering the dose following improvement prevents relapse. |

Source: National Asthma Education and Prevention Program, *Expert Panel Report II: Guidelines for the Diagnosis and Management of Asthma*, National Heart, Lung, and Blood Institute, 1997.

## AEROSOL DELIVERY DEVICES

| Device/Drugs | Population | Optimal Technique | Therapeutic Issues |
|---|---|---|---|
| Metered-dose inhaler (MDI)<br>Beta$_2$-agonist<br>Corticosteroids<br>Cromolyn sodium and nedocromil<br>Anticholinergics | >5 years | Actuation during a slow (30 L/min or 3-5 seconds) deep inhalation, followed by 10-second breath-holding.<br><br>Under laboratory conditions, open mouth technique (holding MDI 2 inches away from open mouth) enhances delivery to the lungs. However, it has not consistently been shown to enhance clinical benefit compared to closed-mouth technique (closing lips around MDI mouthpiece). | Slow inhalation may be difficult. Difficulty with coordination of actuation and inhalation, particularly in young children and elderly. Patients may incorrectly stop inhalation at actuation. Deposition of 80 percent of actuated dose in oropharynx. Mouth washing is effective in reducing systemic absorption. |
| Breath-actuated MDI<br>Beta$_2$-agonists | >5 years | Slow (30 L/min or 3-5 seconds) inhalation followed by 10-second breath-holding. | Indicated for patients unable to coordinate inhalation and actuation. May be particularly useful in elderly. Slow inhalation may be difficult and patients may incorrectly stop inhalation at actuation. Requires more rapid inspiration to activate than is optimal for deposition. Cannot be used with currently available spacer/holding chamber devices. |
| Dry powder inhaler (DPI)<br>Beta$_2$-agonists<br>Corticosteroids | ≥5 years | Rapid (60 L/min or 1-2 seconds), deep inhalation. Minimally effective inspiratory flow is device dependent. | Dose lost if patient exhales through device. Delivery can be ≥ MDI depending on device and technique. Can be used in children 4 years old, but effects are more consistent with children >5. Most appear to have similar delivery efficiency as MDI either with or without spacer/holding chamber, but some may have delivery >MDI. Mouth washing is effective in reducing systemic absorption. |
| Spacer/holding chamber | >4 years<br><br>≤4 years with face mask | Slow (30 L/min or 3-5 seconds) inhalation or tidal breathing immediately following actuation.<br><br>Actuation only once into spacer/holding chamber per inhalation. If face mask is used, allow 3-5 inhalations per actuation. | Easier to use than MDI alone. With a face mask, enables MDI to be used with small children. Simple tubes do not obviate coordinating actuation and inhalation. Bulky. Output may be reduced in some devices after cleaning. The larger volume spacers/holding chambers (>600 cc) may increase lung delivery over MDI alone in patients with poor MDI technique. The effect of a spacer/holding chamber on output from an MDI is dependent on both MDI and spacer type; thus data from one combination should not be extrapolated to all others.<br><br>Spacers/holding chambers decrease oropharyngeal deposition and will reduce potential system absorption of inhaled corticosteroid preparations that have higher oral bioavailability. Spacers/holding chambers are recommended for all patients on medium-to-high doses of inhaled corticosteroids.<br><br>May be as effective as nebulizer in delivering high doses of beta$_2$-agonists during severe exacerbations. |

*continues*

**Aerosol Delivery Devices** continued

| Device/Drugs | Population | Optimal Technique | Therapeutic Issues |
|---|---|---|---|
| Nebulizer<br>Beta$_2$-agonists<br>Cromolyn<br>Anticholinergics<br>Corticosteroids | ≤2 years<br><br>Patients of any age who cannot use MDI with spacer/holding chamber or spacer and face mask (e.g., during exacerbations) | Slow tidal breathing with occasional deep breaths. Tightly fitting face mask for those unable to use mouthpiece. | Less dependent on patient coordination or cooperation.<br><br>Delivery method of choice for cromolyn in children and for high-dose beta$_2$-agonists and anticholinergics in moderate-to-severe exacerbations in all patients.<br><br>Expensive; time consuming; bulky; output is device dependent; and there are significant internebulizer and intranebulizer output variances. |

Source: National Asthma Education and Prevention Program, *Expert Panel Report II: Guidelines for the Diagnosis and Management of Asthma*, National Heart, Lung, and Blood Institute, 1997.

## KEY RECOMMENDATIONS FOR MANAGING ASTHMA LONG TERM

- Persistent asthma is most effectively controlled with daily long-term-control medication, specifically, anti-inflammatory therapy.
- A stepwise approach to pharmacologic therapy is recommended to gain and maintain control of asthma:
  - The amount and frequency of medication is dictated by asthma severity and directed toward suppression of airway inflammation.
  - Therapy should be initiated at a higher level than the patient's step of severity at the onset to establish prompt control and then stepped down.
  - Continual monitoring is essential to ensure that asthma control is achieved.
  - Step-down therapy is essential to identify the minimum medication necessary to maintain control.
- Regular followup visits (at 1- to 6-month intervals) are essential to ensure that control is maintained and the appropriate step down in therapy is considered.
- Therapeutic strategies should be considered in concert with clinician-patient partnership strategies; education of patients is essential for achieving optimal pharmacologic therapy.
- At each step, patients should be advised to avoid or control allergens, irritants, or other factors that make the patient's asthma worse.
- Referral to an asthma specialist for consultation or co-management of the patient is recommended if there are difficulties achieving or maintaining control of asthma or if the patient requires step 4 care. Referral may be considered if the patient requires step 3 care. For infants and young children, referral is recommended if the patient requires step 3 or 4 care and should be considered if the patient requires step 2 care.

Source: National Asthma Education and Prevention Program, *Expert Panel Report II: Guidelines for the Diagnosis and Management of Asthma*, National Heart, Lung, and Blood Institute, 1997.

## GAINING CONTROL OF ASTHMA

The clinician must judge individual patient needs and circumstances to determine at what step to initiate therapy. There are two appropriate approaches to gaining control of asthma:

- Start treatment at the step appropriate to the severity of the patient's disease at the time of evaluation and gradually step up if control is not achieved.

OR

- At the onset, administer therapy at a level higher than the patient's step of severity to gain rapid control. This can be accomplished by either a short course of systemic corticosteroids along with inhaled corticosteroids or initiating a medium-to-high dose of inhaled corticosteroids. Once control is gained, step down the therapy.

**The more aggressive approach of gaining prompt control with a higher level of therapy is preferred, in the opinion of the Expert Panel.**

**Two Approaches To Gaining Control of Asthma: (1) Start with High-Dose Therapy and Step Down or (2) Gradually Step Up Therapy**

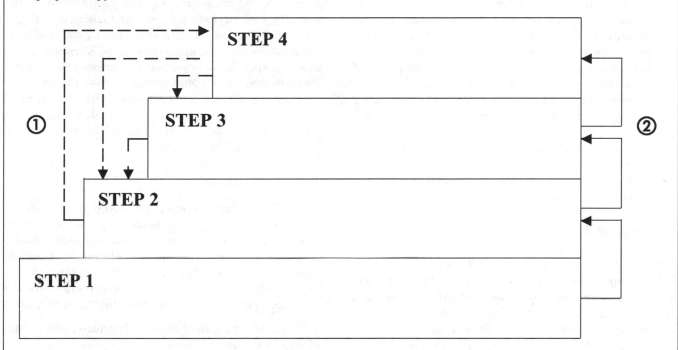

Source: National Asthma Education and Prevention Program, *Expert Panel Report II: Guidelines for the Diagnosis and Management of Asthma*, National Heart, Lung, and Blood Institute, 1997.

## Pharmacologic Steps

The following recommendations for pharmacologic therapy at different steps of asthma severity are intended to be general guidelines for making therapeutic decisions. They are not intended to be prescriptions for individual treatment. Specific therapy should be tailored to the needs and circumstances of individual patients. Pharmacologic therapy must be accompanied at every step by patient education and measures to control those factors that contribute to the severity of the asthma.

If optimal control of asthma is not achieved and sustained at any step of care (nocturnal symptoms, urgent care visits, or an increased need for short-acting beta$_2$-agonists are key indications that asthma is not optimally controlled), several actions may be considered:

- **Patient adherence and technique in using medications correctly should be assessed.**
- **A temporary increase in anti-inflammatory therapy may be indicated to reestablish control.** A deterioration of asthma may be characterized by gradual reduction in PEF (approximately 20 percent), by failure of inhaled bronchodilators to produce a sustained response, by a reduced tolerance to activities or exercise, and by the development of increasing nocturnal symptoms. To regain control of asthma, a short course of oral prednisone is often effective. If asthma symptoms do not recur and pulmonary functions remain normal, no additional therapy is necessary. However, if the prednisone burst does not control symptoms, is effective only for a short period of time (e.g., less than 1 to 2 weeks), or is repeated frequently, the patient should be managed according to the next higher step of care.
- **Other factors that diminish control may need to be identified and addressed.** These factors include the presence of a coexisting condition (e.g., sinusitis), a new or increased exposure to allergens or irritants, patient or family barriers to adequate self-management behaviors, or psychosocial problems. In some cases, alternative diagnoses may need to be considered, such as vocal cord dysfunction.
- **A step up to the next higher step of care may be necessary.**
- **Consultation with an asthma specialist may be indicated.**

## Intermittent Asthma

*Step 1: Mild Intermittent Asthma.* **Short-acting inhaled beta$_2$-agonists taken as needed to treat symptoms are usually sufficient therapy for mild, intermittent asthma.** If effective in relieving symptoms and normalizing pulmonary function, intermittent use of short-acting inhaled beta$_2$-agonists can continue to be used on an as-needed basis. If significant symptoms reoccur or beta$_2$-agonist is required for quick-relief treatment more than two times a week (with the exception of using beta$_2$-agonist for exacerbations caused by viral infections and for exercise-induced bronchospasm [EIB]), the patient should be moved to the next step of care.

Patients with intermittent asthma who experience EIB benefit from taking inhaled beta$_2$-agonists, cromolyn, or nedocromil shortly before exercise. Cromolyn or nedocromil taken before unavoidable exposure to an aeroallergen known to exacerbate the patient's asthma may be beneficial.

**The Expert Panel recommends the following actions for managing exacerbations due to viral respiratory infections, which are especially common in children.** If the symptoms are mild, inhaled beta$_2$-agonist (ever 4 to 6 hours for 24 hours, longer with a physician consult) may be sufficient to control symptoms and improve lung function. If this therapy needs to be repeated more frequently than every 6 weeks, a step up in long-term care is recommended. If the viral respiratory infection provokes a moderate-to-severe exacerbation, a short course of systemic corticosteroids should be considered. For those patients with a history of severe exacerbations with viral respiratory infections, systemic corticosteroids should be initiated at the first sign of the infection.

**The Expert Panel recommends that a detailed written action plan be developed for those patients with intermittent asthma who have a history of severe exacerbations.** Intermittent asthma—infrequent exacerbations separated by periods of no symptoms and normal pulmonary function—is often mild. However, some patients with intermittent asthma experience sudden, severe, and life-threatening exacerbations. It is essential to treat these exacerbations accordingly. The patient's action plan should include indicators of worsening asthma (specific symptoms and PEF measurements), as well as specific recommendations for using beta$_2$-agonist rescue therapy, early administration of systemic corticosteroids, and seeking medical care. Furthermore, periodic monitoring of the patient is appropriate to evaluate whether the patient's asthma is indeed intermittent or whether a step up in long-term therapy is warranted.

## Persistent Asthma

**The Expert Panel recommends that patients with persistent asthma, either mild, moderate, or severe, receive daily long-term-control medication. The most effective long-term-control medications are those with anti-inflammatory effects, that is, those that diminish chronic airway inflammation and airway hyperresponsiveness.** Evidence from clinical trials supports this recommendation.

*Step 2: Mild Persistent Asthma.* The main characteristics of Step 2 care are as follows:

- **Step 2 care long-term-control medication is daily anti-inflammatory medication: either inhaled corticosteroids at a low dose, cromolyn, or nedocromil.** For children, a trial of cromolyn or nedocromil is often the initial long-term therapy due to the safety profiles of these medications.
- **Sustained-release theophylline is an alternative, but not preferred, long-term-control medication.** It is not preferred because its modest clinical effectiveness (theophylline is primarily a bronchodilator and its anti-inflammatory activity demonstrated thus far is modest) must be balanced against concerns about potential toxicity. Theophylline remains a therapeutic option for

certain patients due to expense or need for tablet-form medication. Sustained-release theophylline is given to achieve a serum concentration of between 5 and 15 mcg/ mL. Periodic theophylline monitoring is necessary to maintain a therapeutic—but not toxic—level.

- **Zafirlukast or zileuton may also be considered an alternative long-term-control medication for patients older than 12 years of age, although their position in therapy is not yet fully established.** Initial experience in clinical trials and possible patient requirements for tablet-form medication make these new medications a therapeutic option. Further clinical experience and additional data are needed to establish the role of zafirlukast and zileuton in stepwise therapy.

- **Quick-relief medication must be available. Inhaled short-acting beta$_2$-agonists should be taken as needed to relieve symptoms.** The intensity of treatment will depend on the severity of the exacerbation. Use of inhaled short-acting beta$_2$-agonists on a daily basis, or increasing use, indicates the need for additional long-term-control therapy.

*Step 3: Moderate Persistent Asthma.* Consultation with an asthma specialist may be considered because the therapeutic options at this juncture pose a number of challenging risk/benefit outcomes. There are at least three options for initiating Step 3 therapy.

- **Increase inhaled corticosteroids to medium dose.** This strategy will benefit many patients. Adverse effects, although infrequent, may arise (see component 3—Medications).

OR

- **Add a long-acting bronchodilator to a low-to-medium dose of inhaled corticosteroids.** The long-acting bronchodilator may be either a long-acting inhaled beta$_2$-agonist (e.g., salmeterol) or sustained-release theophylline; although not preferred, long-acting beta$_2$-agonist tablets may be considered. This approach has been shown to improve symptom control and may be especially beneficial in patients who have significant nocturnal symptoms. Improved asthma control has been demonstrated with an inhaled long-acting beta$_2$-agonist and a medium-dose inhaled corticosteroid compared to a doubled dose of inhaled corticosteroid, but the potential for incorrectly using long-acting inhaled beta$_2$-agonists as a quick-relief medication needs to be considered. The approach of adding theophylline

has the potential for adverse reactions related to fluctuations in theophylline serum concentrations.

OR

- **Establish control with medium-dose inhaled corticosteroids, then lower the dose (but still within the medium-dose range) and add nedocromil.** Nedocromil has a notable safety profile, and some studies have shown that it has some, albeit modest, inhaled corticosteroid-sparing effects in adults. Other studies did not demonstrate this. Therefore, this treatment option is not preferred. Furthermore, adding another inhaler into the patient's medication schedule may affect patient adherence. It will also affect the total cost of care.

**If the patient's asthma is not optimally controlled with initial Step 3 therapy, and medications are used correctly, additional Step 3 therapy is recommended.**

- **Increase daily long-term-control medications to a high dose of inhaled corticosteroids,**

AND

- **Add a long-acting bronchodilator**, especially to control nocturnal symptoms. The long-acting bronchodilator can be either long-acting inhaled beta$_2$-agonist or sustained-release theophylline. An evening dose of either bronchodilator may alleviate and prevent nocturnal symptoms and thus improve adherence to the overall therapeutic regimen.

*Step 4: Severe Persistent Asthma.* **Patients whose asthma is not controlled on high doses of inhaled corticosteroids and the addition of long-acting bronchodilators will also need oral systemic corticosteroids on a regularly scheduled, long-term basis.** For patients who require long-term systemic corticosteroids:

- Use the lowest possible dose (single dose daily or on alternate days).
- Monitor patients closely for corticosteroid adverse side effects.
- When control of asthma is achieved, make persistent attempts to reduce systemic corticosteroids. High doses of inhaled corticosteroids are preferable to systemic corticosteroids because inhaled corticosteroids have fewer systemic effects.
- Consultation with an asthma specialist is recommended.

## SPECIAL CONSIDERATIONS FOR MANAGING ASTHMA IN DIFFERENT AGE GROUPS—KEY RECOMMENDATIONS

### INFANTS AND YOUNG CHILDREN (5 YEARS OF AGE AND YOUNGER)

- Diagnosing asthma in infants is often difficult, yet under-diagnosis and undertreatment are key problems in this age group. Thus, a diagnostic trial of inhaled bronchodilators and anti-inflammatory medications may be helpful.
- In general, infants and young children consistently requiring symptomatic treatment more than two times per week should be given daily anti-inflammatory therapy.
- When initiating daily anti-inflammatory therapy, a trial of cromolyn or nedocromil is often given due to the safety profile of these medications.
- Response to therapy should be carefully monitored. Once control of asthma symptoms is established and sustained, a careful step down in therapy should be attempted. If clear benefit is not observed, alternative therapies or diagnoses should be considered.

### SCHOOL-AGE CHILDREN (OLDER THAN 5 YEARS OF AGE) AND ADOLESCENTS

- Pulmonary function testing should use appropriate reference populations. Adolescents compare better to childhood than to adult predicted norms.
- When initiating daily anti-inflammatory therapy for mild-to-moderate persistent asthma, a trial of cromolyn or nedocromil is often given.
- Adolescents (and younger children as appropriate) should be directly involved in establishing goals for therapy and developing their asthma management plans.
- Active participation in physical activities, exercise, and sports should be promoted.
- A written asthma management plan should be prepared for the student's school, including plans to ensure reliable, prompt access to medications.

### OLDER ADULTS

- Chronic bronchitis/emphysema may coexist with asthma. A trial of systemic corticosteroids will determine the presence of reversibility and the extent of therapeutic benefit.
- Asthma medications may aggravate coexisting medical conditions (e.g., cardiac disease, osteoporosis); adjustments in the medication plan may need to be made.
- Be aware of increased potential for adverse drug/disease interaction (e.g., aspirin, beta-blockers).
- Review of patient technique in using medications and devices is essential.

### Potential Adverse Effects of Medications

Asthma medications may have increased adverse effects in the elderly patient; adjustments in the medication plan may be necessary.

- Airway response to **bronchodilators** may change with age, although this is not clearly established. Older patients, especially those with preexisting ischemic heart disease, may also be more sensitive to beta$_2$-agonist side effects, including tremor and tachycardia. Concomitant use of anticholinergics and beta$_2$-agonists may be beneficial to the older patient.
- **Theophylline** clearance is reduced in the elderly patient, causing increased blood levels of theophylline. In addition, age is an independent risk factor for developing life-threatening events from iatrogenic chronic theophylline overdose (patients 75 years of age or older have a 16-fold greater risk of death from theophylline overdose than do 25-year-olds). The potential for drug interaction—especially with antibiotics and H$_2$-histamine antagonists such as cimetidine—is greater because of the increased use of medications in this age group. Theophylline and epinephrine may exacerbate underlying heart conditions.
- **Systemic corticosteroids** can provoke confusion, agitation, and changes in glucose metabolism.
- A dose-dependent reduction in bone mineral content may be associated with **inhaled corticosteroid** use, although low or medium doses appear to have no major adverse effect. Elderly patients may be more at risk due to preexisting osteoporosis, changes in estrogen levels that affect calcium utilization, and a sedentary lifestyle. However, the risk of not adequately controlling asthma may unnecessarily limit the patient's mobility and activities. **Concurrent treatment with calcium supplements and vitamin D, and estrogen replacement when appropriate, are recommended.** At the present time, the optimal approach for identifying patients at risk for accelerated bone loss from high-dose corticosteroid therapy is to conduct bone densitometry when treatment begins and again 6 months later, although the benefits of this approach have not yet been evaluated in clinical trials.

**Medications employed for other diseases may exacerbate asthma; adjustments may need to be made.** Nonsteroidal anti-inflammatory agents for treating arthritis, nonselective beta-blockers for treating hypertension, or beta-blockers found in some eye drops used to treat glaucoma may exacerbate asthma.

Source: National Asthma Education and Prevention Program, *Expert Panel Report II: Guidelines for the Diagnosis and Management of Asthma*, National Heart, Lung, and Blood Institute, 1997.

# STEPWISE APPROACH FOR MANAGING ASTHMA IN ADULTS AND CHILDREN OLDER THAN 5 YEARS OF AGE: TREATMENT

**Note: Preferred treatments are in bold print.**

| | Long-Term Control | Quick Relief | Education |
|---|---|---|---|
| **STEP 4**<br>Severe Persistent | Daily medications:<br>• **Anti-inflammatory: inhaled corticosteroid (high dose) AND**<br>• Long-acting bronchodilator: either **long-acting inhaled beta$_2$-agonist**, sustained-release theophylline, or long-acting beta$_2$-agonist tablets AND<br>• Corticosteroid tablets or syrup long term (2 mg/kg/day, generally do not exceed 60 mg per day). | • Short-acting bronchodilator: **inhaled beta$_2$-agonists** as needed for symptoms.<br>• Intensity of treatment will depend on severity of exacerbation.<br>• Use of short-acting inhaled beta$_2$-agonists on a daily basis, or increasing use, indicates the need for additional long-term-control therapy. | Steps 2 and 3 actions plus:<br>• Refer to individual education/counseling |
| **STEP 3**<br>Moderate Persistent | Daily medication:<br>• Either<br>  –**Anti-inflammatory: inhaled corticosteroid (medium dose)**<br>  OR<br>  –**Inhaled corticosteroid (low–medium dose)** and add a long-acting bronchodilator, especially for nighttime symptoms: either **long-acting inhaled beta$_2$-agonist**, sustained-release theophylline, or long-acting beta$_2$-agonist tablets.<br>• If needed<br>  –**Anti-inflammatory: inhaled corticosteroids (medium–high dose) AND**<br>  –**Long-acting bronchodilator**, especially for nighttime symptoms; either **long-acting inhaled beta$_2$-agonist**, sustained-release theophylline, or long-acting beta$_2$-agonist tablets. | • Short-acting bronchodilator: **inhaled beta$_2$-agonists** as needed for symptoms.<br>• Intensity of treatment will depend on severity of exacerbation.<br>• Use of short-acting inhaled beta$_2$-agonists on a daily basis, or increasing use, indicates the need for additional long-term-control therapy. | Step 1 actions plus:<br>• Teach self-monitoring<br>• Refer to group education if available<br>• Review and update self-management plan |
| **STEP 2**<br>Mild Persistent | One daily medication:<br>• **Anti-inflammatory:** either **inhaled corticosteroid** (low doses) or **cromolyn or nedocromil** (children usually begin with a trial of cromolyn or nedocromil).<br>• Sustained-release theophylline to serum concentration of 5-15 mcg/mL is an alternative, but not preferred, therapy. Zafirlukast or zileuton may also be considered for patients ≥12 years of age, although their position in therapy is not fully established. | • Short-acting bronchodilator: **inhaled beta$_2$-agonists** as needed for symptoms.<br>• Intensity of treatment will depend on severity of exacerbation.<br>• Use of short-acting inhaled beta$_2$-agonists on a daily basis, or increasing use, indicates the need for additional long-term-control therapy. | Step 1 actions plus:<br>• Teach self-monitoring<br>• Refer to group education if available<br>• Review and update self-management plan |

*continues*

**Stepwise Approach for Managing Asthma in Adults and Children Older Than 5 Years of Age: Treatment** continued

**Note: Preferred treatments are in bold print.**

| | Long-Term Control | Quick Relief | Education |
|---|---|---|---|
| **STEP 1**<br>**Mild**<br>**Intermittent** | • No daily medication needed. | • Short-acting bronchodilator: **inhaled beta$_2$-agonists** as needed for symptoms.<br>• Intensity of treatment will depend on severity of exacerbation; see component 3—Managing Exacerbations.<br>• Use of short-acting inhaled beta$_2$-agonists more than 2 times a week may indicate the need to initiate long-term-control therapy. | • Teach basic facts about asthma<br>• Teach inhaler/spacer/holder chamber technique<br>• Discuss roles of medications<br>• Develop self-management plan<br>• Develop action plan for when and how to take rescue actions, especially for patients with a history of severe exacerbations<br>• Discuss appropriate environmental control measures to avoid exposure to known allergens and irritants |

↓ **Step down**

Review treatment every 1 to 6 months; a gradual stepwise reduction in treatment may be possible.

↑ **Step up**

If control is not maintained, consider step up. First, review patient medication technique, adherence, and environmental control (avoidance of allergens or other factors that contribute to asthma severity).

**NOTES:**
• **The stepwise approach presents general guidelines to assist clinical decisionmaking; it is not intended to be a specific prescription. Asthma is highly variable; clinicians should tailor specific medication plans to the needs and circumstances of individual patients.**
• Gain control as quickly as possible; then decrease treatment to the least medication necessary to maintain control. Gaining control may be accomplished by either starting treatment at the step most appropriate to the initial severity of the condition or starting at a higher level of therapy (e.g., a course of systemic corticosteroids or higher dose of inhaled corticosteroids).
• A rescue course of systemic corticosteroids may be needed at any time and at any step.
• Some patients with intermittent asthma experience severe and life-threatening exacerbations separated by long periods of normal lung function and no symptoms. This may be especially common with exacerbations provoked by respiratory infections. A short course of systemic corticosteroids is recommended.
• At each step, patients should control their environment to avoid or control factors that make their asthma worse (e.g., allergens, irritants); this requires specific diagnosis and education.

Source: National Asthma Education and Prevention Program, *Expert Panel Report II: Guidelines for the Diagnosis and Management of Asthma*, National Heart, Lung, and Blood Institute, 1997.

## USUAL DOSAGES FOR LONG-TERM CONTROL MEDICATIONS

| Medication | Dosage Form | Adult Dose | Child Dose | Comments |
|---|---|---|---|---|
| **Inhaled Corticosteroids** | See exhibit titled "Estimated Comparative Daily Dosages for Inhaled Corticosteroids" on p. 69 for dosage information on inhaled corticosteroids. | | | |
| **Systemic Corticosteroids** | | (Applies to all three systemic corticosteroids) | | |
| Methylprednisolone | 2, 4, 8, 16, 32 mg tablets | | | • For long-term treatment of severe persistent asthma, administer single dose in a.m. either daily or on alternate days (alternate-day therapy may produce less adrenal suppression). If daily doses are required, one study suggests improved efficacy at no increase in adrenal suppression when administered at 3:00 p.m. |
| Prednisolone | 5 mg tablets, 5 mg/cc, 15 mg/cc | • 7.5-60 mg daily in a single dose or qid as needed for control<br>• Short-course "burst": 40-60 mg per day as single or 2 divided doses for 3-10 days | • 0.25-2 mg/kg daily in single dose or qid as needed for control<br>• Short course "burst": 1-2 mg/kg/day, maximum 60 mg/day, for 3-10 days | • Short courses or "bursts" are effective for establishing control when initiating therapy or during a period of gradual deterioration. |
| Prednisone | 1, 2.5, 5, 10, 20, 25 mg tablets; 5 mg/cc solution | | | • The burst should be continued until patient achieves 80% PEF personal best or symptoms resolve. This usually requires 3-10 days but may require longer. There is no evidence that tapering the dose following improvement prevents relapse. |
| **Cromolyn and Nedocromil** | | | | |
| Cromolyn | MDI 1 mg/puff<br>Nebulizer solution 20 mg/ampule | 2-4 puffs tid-qid<br>1 ampule tid-qid | 1-2 puffs tid-qid<br>1 ampule tid-qid | • One dose prior to exercise or allergen exposure provides effective prophylaxis for 1-2 hours. |
| Nedocromil | MDI 1.75 mg/puff | 2-4 puffs bid-qid | 1-2 puffs bid-qid | • See cromolyn above. |
| **Long-Acting Beta₂-Agonists** | | | | |
| Salmeterol | **Inhaled**<br>MDI 21 mcg/puff, 60 or 120 puffs<br>DPI 50 mcg/blister | 2 puffs q 12 hours<br>1 blister q 12 hours | 1-2 puffs q 12 hours<br>1 blister q 12 hours | • May use one dose nightly for symptoms.<br>• **Should not be used for symptom relief or for exacerbations.** |
| Sustained-Release Albuterol | **Tablet**<br>4 mg tablet | 4 mg q 12 hours | 0.3-0.6 mg/kg/day, not to exceed 8 mg/day | |
| **Methylxanthines** | | | | |
| Theophylline | Liquids, sustained-release tablets, and capsules | Starting dose 10 mg/kg/day up to 300 mg max; usual max 800 mg/day | Starting dose 10 mg/kg/day; usual max:<br>• <1 year of age: 0.2 (age in weeks) + 5 = mg/kg/day<br>• ≥1 year of age: 16 mg/kg/day | • Adjust dosage to achieve serum concentration of 5-15 mcg/mL at steady-state (at least 48 hours on same dosage).<br>• Due to wide interpatient variability in theophylline metabolic clearance, **routine serum theophylline level monitoring is important.**<br>• See factors below that can affect levels. |

*continues*

**Usual Dosages for Long-Term Control Medications** continued

### Factors Affecting Serum Theophylline Concentrations*

| Factor | Decreases Theophylline Concentrations (↓ or delays absorption of some sustained-release theophylline (SRT) products) | Increases Theophylline Concentrations (↑ rate of absorption (fatty foods) products) | Recommended Action |
|---|---|---|---|
| Food | | | Select theophylline preparation that is not affected by food. |
| Diet | ↑ metabolism (high protein) | ↑ metabolism (high carbohydrate) | Inform patients that major changes in diet are not recommended while taking theophylline. |
| Systemic, febrile viral illness (e.g., influenza) | | ↓ metabolism | Decrease theophylline dose according to serum concentration level. Decrease dose by 50 percent if serum concentration measurement is not available. |
| Hypoxia, cor pulmonale, and decompensated congestive heart failure, cirrhosis | | ↓ metabolism | Decrease dose according to serum concentration level. |
| Age | ↑ metabolism (1 to 9 years) | ↓ metabolism (<6 months, elderly) | Adjust dose according to serum concentration level. |
| Phenobarbital, phenytoin, carbamazepine | ↑ metabolism | | Increase dose according to serum concentration level. |
| Cimetidine | | ↓ metabolism | Use alternative $H_2$ blocker (e.g., famotidine or ranitidine). |
| Macrolides: TAO, erythromycin, clarithromycin | | ↓ metabolism | Use alternative antibiotic or adjust theophylline dose. |
| Quinolones: ciprofloxacin, enoxacin, pefloxacin | | ↓ metabolism | Use alternative antibiotic or adjust theophylline dose. Circumvent with ofloxacin if quinolone therapy is required. |
| Rifampin | ↑ metabolism | | Increase dose according to serum concentration level. |
| Ticlopidine | | ↓ metabolism | Decrease dose according to serum concentration level. |
| Smoking | ↑ metabolism | | Advise patient to stop smoking; increase dose according to serum concentration level. |
| *Leukotriene Modifiers* | | | |
| Zafirlukast | 20 mg tablet | 40 mg daily (1 tablet bid) | • For zafirlukast, administration with meals decreases bioavailability; take at least 1 hour before or 2 hours after meals. |
| Zileuton | 300 mg tablet 600 mg tablet | 2,400 mg daily (two 300 mg tablets or one 600 mg tablet, qid) | • For zileuton, monitor hepatic enzymes (ALT). |

*This list is not all inclusive; for discussion of other factors, see package inserts.

Source: National Asthma Education and Prevention Program, *Expert Panel Report II: Guidelines for the Diagnosis and Management of Asthma*, National Heart, Lung, and Blood Institute, 1997.

## ESTIMATED COMPARATIVE DAILY DOSAGES FOR INHALED CORTICOSTEROIDS

### ADULTS

| Drug | Low Dose | Medium Dose | High Dose |
|---|---|---|---|
| Beclomethasone dipropionate 42 mcg/puff 84 mcg/puff | 168-504 mcg (4-12 puffs—42 mcg) (2-6 puffs—84 mcg) | 504-840 mcg (12-20 puffs—42 mcg) (6-10 puffs—84 mcg) | >840 mcg (>20 puffs—42 mcg) (>10 puffs—84 mcg) |
| Budesonide Turbuhaler 200 mcg/dose | 200-400 mcg (1-2 inhalations) | 400-600 mcg (2-3 inhalations) | >600 mcg (>3 inhalations) |
| Flunisolide 250 mcg/puff | 500-1,000 mcg (2-4 puffs) | 1,000-2,000 mcg (4-8 puffs) | >2,000 mcg (>8 puffs) |
| Fluticasone MDI: 44, 110, 220 mcg/puff DPI: 50, 100, 250 mcg/dose | 88-264 mcg (2-6 puffs—44 mcg) or (2 puffs—110 mcg) (2-6 inhalations—50 mcg) | 264-660 mcg (2-6 puffs—110 mcg) (3-6 inhalations—100 mcg) | >660 mcg (>6 puffs—110 mcg) or (>3 puffs—220 mcg) (>6 inhalations—100 mcg) |
| Triamcinolone acetonide 100 mcg/puff | 400-1,000 mcg (4-10 puffs) | 1,000-2,000 mcg (10-20 puffs) | >2,000 mcg (>20 puffs) |

### CHILDREN

| Drug | Low Dose | Medium Dose | High Dose |
|---|---|---|---|
| Beclomethasone dipropionate 42 mcg/puff 84 mcg/puff | 84-336 mcg (2-8 puffs) | 336-672 mcg (8-16 puffs) | >672 mcg (>16 puffs) |
| Budesonide Turbuhaler 200 mcg/dose | 100-200 mcg | 200-400 mcg (1-2 inhalations—200 mcg) | >400 mcg (>2 inhalations—200 mcg) |
| Flunisolide 250 mcg/puff | 500-750 mcg (2-3 puffs) | 1,000-1,250 mcg (4-5 puffs) | >1,250 mcg (>5 puffs) |
| Fluticasone MDI: 44, 110, 220 mcg/puff DPI: 50, 100, 250 mcg/dose | 88-176 mcg (2-4 puffs—44 mcg) (2-4 inhalations—50 mcg) | 176-440 mcg (4-10 puffs—44 mcg) or (2 puffs—110 mcg) (2-4 inhalations—100 mcg) | >440 mcg (>4 puffs—110 mcg) (>4 inhalations—100 mcg) |
| Triamcinolone acetonide 100 mcg/puff | 400-800 mcg (4-8 puffs) | 800-1,200 mcg (8-12 puffs) | >1,200 mcg (>12 puffs) |

### NOTES:

- **The most important determinant of appropriate dosing is the clinician's judgment of the patient's response to therapy.** The clinician must monitor the patient's response on several clinical parameters and adjust the dose accordingly. The stepwise approach to therapy emphasizes that once control of asthma is achieved, the dose of medication should be carefully titrated to the minimum dose required to maintain control, thus reducing the potential for adverse effect.
- The reference point for the range in the dosages for children is data on the safety of inhaled corticosteroids in children, which, in general, suggest that the dose ranges are equivalent to beclomethasone dipropionate 200-400 mcg/day (low dose), 400-800 mcg/day (medium dose), and >800 mcg/day (high dose).
- Some dosages may be outside package labeling.
- Metered-dose inhaler (MDI) dosages are expressed as the actuater dose (the amount of drug leaving the actuater and delivered to the patient), which is the labeling required in the United States. This is different from the dosage expressed as the valve dose (the amount of drug leaving the valve, all of which is not available to the patient), which is used in many European countries and in some of the scientific literature. Dry powder inhaler (DPI) doses (e.g., Turbuhaler) are expressed as the amount of drug in the inhaler following activation.

Source: National Asthma Education and Prevention Program, *Expert Panel Report II: Guidelines for the Diagnosis and Management of Asthma*, National Heart, Lung, and Blood Institute, 1997.

## USUAL DOSAGES FOR QUICK-RELIEF MEDICATIONS

| Medication | Dosage Form | Adult Dose | Child Dose | Comments |
|---|---|---|---|---|
| **Short-Acting Inhaled Beta₂-Agonists** | | | | |
| | *MDIs* | | | • An increasing use or lack of expected effect indicates diminished control of asthma. |
| Albuterol | 90 mcg/puff, 200 puffs | • 2 puffs q 5 minutes prior to exercise | • 1-2 puffs 5 minutes prior to exercise | • Not generally recommended for long-term treatment. Regular use on a daily basis indicates the need for additional long-term-control therapy. |
| Albuterol HFA | 90 mcg/puff, 200 puffs | • 2 puffs tid-qid prn | • 2 puffs tid-qid prn | • Differences in potency exist so that all products are essentially equipotent on a per-puff basis. |
| Bitolterol | 370 mcg/puff, 300 puffs | | | • May double usual dose for mild exacerbations. |
| Pirbuterol | 200 mcg/puff, 400 puffs | | | • Nonselective agents (i.e., epinephrine, isoproterenol, metaproterenol) are not recommended. |
| Terbutaline | 200 mcg/puff, 300 puffs | | | |
| | *DPI* | | | |
| Albuterol Rotahaler | 200 mcg/capsule | 1-2 capsules q 4-6 hours as needed and prior to exercise | 1 capsule q 4-6 hours as needed and prior to exercise | |
| | *Nebulizer solution* | | | |
| Albuterol | 5 mg/mL (0.5%) | 1.25-5 mg (.25-1 cc) in 2-3 cc of saline q 4-8 hours | 0.05 mg/kg (min 1.25 mg, max 2.5 mg) in 2-3 cc of saline q 4-6 hours | May mix with cromolyn or ipratropium nebulizer solutions. May double dose for mild exacerbations. |
| Bitolterol | 2 mg/mL (0.2%) | 0.5-3.5 mg (.25-1 cc) in 2-3 cc of saline q 4-8 hours | Not established | May not mix with other nebulizer solutions. |
| **Anticholinergics** | | | | |
| | *MDI* | | | Evidence is lacking for anticholinergics producing added benefit to beta₂-agonists in long-term asthma therapy. |
| Ipratropium | 18 mcg/puff, 200 puffs | 2-3 puffs q 6 hours | 1-2 puffs q 6 hours | |
| | *Nebulizer solution* | | | |
| | .25 mg/mL (0.025%) | 0.25-0.5 mg q 6 hours | 0.25 mg q 6 hours | |
| **Systemic Corticosteroids** | | (Applies to all three systemic corticosteroids) | | |
| Methylprednisolone | 2, 4, 8, 16, 32 mg tablets | • Short course "burst": 40-60 mg/day as single or 2 divided doses for 3-10 days | • Short course "burst": 1-2 mg/kg/day, maximum 60 mg/day, for 3-10 days | • Short courses or "bursts" are effective for establishing control when initiating therapy or during a period of gradual deterioration. |
| Prednisolone | 5 mg tabs, 5 mg/cc, 15 mg/cc | | | • The burst should be continued until patient achieves 80% PEF personal best or symptoms resolve. This usually requires 3-10 days but may require longer. There is no evidence that tapering the dose following improvement prevents relapse. |
| Prednisone | 1, 2.5, 5, 10, 20, 25 mg tabs; 5 mg/cc solution | | | |

Source: National Asthma Education and Prevention Program, *Expert Panel Report II: Guidelines for the Diagnosis and Management of Asthma*, National Heart, Lung, and Blood Institute, 1997.

## STEPWISE APPROACH FOR MANAGING INFANTS AND YOUNG CHILDREN (5 YEARS OF AGE AND YOUNGER) WITH ACUTE OR CHRONIC ASTHMA SYMPTOMS

| | Long-Term Control | Quick Relief |
|---|---|---|
| **STEP 4** Severe Persistent | • Daily anti-inflammatory medicine <br> – High-dose inhaled corticosteroid with spacer/holding chamber and face mask <br> – If needed, add systemic corticosteroids 2 mg/kg/day and reduce to lowest daily or alternate-day dose that stabilizes symptoms | • Bronchodilator as needed for symptoms (see step 1) up to 3 times a day |
| **STEP 3** Moderate Persistent | • Daily anti-inflammatory medication. Either: <br> – Medium-dose inhaled corticosteroid with spacer/holding chamber and face mask <br>     OR, once control is established: <br> – Medium-dose inhaled corticosteroid and nedocromil <br>     OR <br> – Medium-dose inhaled corticosteroid and long-acting bronchodilator (theophylline) | • Bronchodilator as needed for symptoms (see step 1) up to 3 times a day |
| **STEP 2** Mild Persistent | • Daily anti-inflammatory medication. Either: <br> – Cromolyn (nebulizer is preferred; or MDI) or nedocromil (MDI only) tid-qid <br> – Infants and young children usually begin with a trial of cromolyn or nedocromil <br>     OR <br> – Low-dose inhaled corticosteroid with spacer/holding chamber and face mask | • Bronchodilator as needed for symptoms (see step 1) |
| **STEP 1** Mild Intermittent | • No daily medication needed | • Bronchodilator as needed for symptoms <2 times a week. Intensity of treatment will depend upon severity of exacerbation. Either: <br> – Inhaled short-acting beta$_2$-agonist by nebulizer or face mask and spacer/holding chamber <br>     OR <br> – Oral beta$_2$-agonist for symptoms <br> • With viral respiratory infection: <br> – Bronchodilator q 4-6 hours up to 24 hours (longer with physician consult) but, in general, repeat no more than once every 6 weeks <br> – Consider systemic corticosteroid if <br>   –Current exacerbation is severe <br>     OR <br>   –Patient has history of previous severe exacerbations |

*continues*

**Stepwise Approach for Managing Infants and Young Children** continued

NOTES:

- **The stepwise approach presents guidelines to assist clinical decision making. Asthma is highly variable; clinicians should tailor specific medication plans to the needs and circumstances of individual patients.**
- Gain control as quickly as possible; then decrease treatment to the least medication necessary to maintain control. Gaining control may be accomplished by either starting treatment at the step most appropriate to the initial severity of the condition or by starting at a higher level of therapy (e.g., a course of systemic corticosteroids or higher dose of inhaled corticosteroids).
- A rescue course of systemic corticosteroid (prednisolone) may be needed at any time and step.
- In general, use of short-acting beta$_2$-agonist on a daily basis indicates the need for additional long-term-control therapy.
- It is important to remember that there are very few studies on asthma therapy for infants.
- Consultation with an asthma specialist is *recommended* for patients with moderate or severe persistent asthma in this age group. Consultation should be *considered* for all patients with mild persistent asthma.

↓ **Step down**
Review treatment every 1 to 6 months. If control is sustained for at least 3 months, a gradual stepwise reduction in treatment may be possible.

↑ **Step up**
If control is not achieved, consider step up. But first: review patient medication technique, adherence, and environmental control (avoidance of allergens or other precipitant factors).

Source: National Asthma Education and Prevention Program, *Expert Panel Report II: Guidelines for the Diagnosis and Management of Asthma*, National Heart, Lung, and Blood Institute, 1997.

# MANAGING SPECIAL SITUATIONS IN ASTHMA*

## Seasonal Asthma

Some patients experience asthma symptoms only in relationship to certain pollens and molds. Such seasonal asthma should be treated according to the stepwise approach to long-term management of asthma. If the patient has seasonal asthma on a predictable basis, daily, long-term anti-inflammatory therapy (inhaled corticosteroids, cromolyn, or nedocromil) should be initiated prior to the anticipated onset of symptoms and continued through the season.

## Cough Variant Asthma

Cough variant asthma is seen especially in young children. Cough is the principal symptom; because this frequently occurs at night, examinations during the day may be normal. Monitoring of morning and afternoon PEF variability and/or therapeutic trials with anti-inflammatory or bronchodilator medication may be helpful in diagnosis. Once the diagnosis is established, treat according to the stepwise approach to long-term management of asthma.

## Exercise-Induced Bronchospasm

Exercise-induced bronchospasm (EIB)—which untreated can limit and disrupt otherwise normal lives—should be anticipated in all asthma patients. EIB is a bronchospastic event that is caused by a loss of heat, water, or both from the lung during exercise because of hyperventilation of air that is cooler and dryer than that of the respiratory tree. EIB usually occurs during or minutes after vigorous activity, reaches its peak 5 to 10 minutes after stopping the activity, and usually resolves in another 20 to 30 minutes.

Exercise may be the only precipitant of asthma symptoms for some patients. These patients should be monitored regularly to ensure that they have no symptoms of asthma or reductions in PEF in the absence of exercise, because EIB is often a marker of inadequate asthma management and responds well to regular anti-inflammatory therapy.

### Diagnosis

A history of cough, shortness of breath, chest pain or tightness, wheezing, or endurance problems during exercise suggests EIB. An exercise challenge can be used to establish the diagnosis. This can be performed in a formal laboratory setting or as a free-run challenge sufficiently strenuous to increase the baseline heart rate to 80 percent of maximum for 4 to 6 minutes. Alternatively, the patient may simply undertake the task that previously caused the symptoms. A 15 percent decrease in PEF or $FEV_1$ (measurements taken before and after exercise at 5-minute intervals for 20 to 30 minutes) is compatible with EIB.

### Management Strategies

One goal of management is to enable patients to participate in any activity they choose without experiencing asthma symptoms. EIB should not limit either participation or success in vigorous activities. **Recommended treatments include:**

- **Beta$_2$-agonists** will prevent EIB in more than 80 percent of patients.
  - Short-acting inhaled beta$_2$-agonists used shortly before exercise (or as close to exercise as possible) may be helpful for 2 to 3 hours.
  - Salmeterol has been shown to prevent EIB for 10 to 12 hours.
- **Cromolyn and nedocromil,** taken shortly before exercise, are also acceptable for preventing EIB.
- **A lengthy warmup period before exercise** may benefit patients who can tolerate continuous exercise with minimal symptoms. The warmup may preclude a need for repeated medications.
- **Long-term-control therapy, if appropriate.** There is evidence that appropriate long-term control of asthma with anti-inflammatory medication will reduce airway responsiveness, and this is associated with a reduction in the frequency and severity of EIB.

**Teachers and coaches need to be notified that a child has EIB,** should be able to participate in activities, and may need inhaled medication before activity.

## Surgery and Asthma

Asthma patients are at risk for specific complications during and after surgery: acute bronchoconstriction triggered by intubation, hypoxemia and possible hypercapnia, impaired effectiveness of cough, atelectasis and respiratory infection, and latex exposure. The likelihood of these complications depends on the severity of the patient's airway hyperresponsiveness, airflow obstruction, mucus hypersecretions, and latex sensitivity.

---

*Source: National Asthma Education and Prevention Program, *Expert Panel Report II: Guidelines for the Diagnosis and Management of Asthma,* National Heart, Lung, and Blood Institute, 1997.

Recommended actions include:

- **Patients with asthma should have an evaluation before surgery that includes a review of symptoms, medication use** (particularly the use of systemic corticosteroids for longer than 2 weeks in the past 6 months), **and measurement of pulmonary function.**
- **If possible, attempts should be made to improve lung function** (FEV$_1$ or PEF) to their predicted values or their personal best level. A short course of systemic corticosteroids may be necessary to optimize pulmonary function.
- **For patients who have received systemic corticosteroids during the past 6 months, give 100 mg hydrocortisone every 8 hours intravenously during the surgical period and reduce dose rapidly within 24 hours following surgery.**

## Pregnancy and Asthma

**Maintaining sufficient lung function and blood oxygenation to ensure adequate oxygen supply to the fetus is essential.** Poorly controlled asthma during pregnancy can result in increased perinatal mortality, increased prematurity, and low birth weight. For most drugs used to treat asthma and rhinitis, with the exception of brompheniramine, epinephrine, and alpha-adrenergic compounds (other than pseudoephedrine), there is little to suggest an increased risk to the fetus. Other classes of drugs with some possibility of risk to the fetus include decongestants (other than pseudoephedrine), antibiotics (tetracycline, sulfonamides, and ciprofloxacin), live virus vaccines, immunotherapy (if doses are increased), and iodides.

## Stress and Asthma

The role of stress and psychological factors in asthma is important but not fully defined. There is emerging evidence that stress can play an important role in precipitating exacerbations of asthma and possibly act as a risk factor for an increase in prevalence of asthma. The mechanisms involved in this process have yet to be fully established and may involve enhanced generation of proinflammatory cytokines. Equally important are psychosocial factors that are associated with poor outcome (e.g., conflict between patients and family and the medical staff, inappropriate asthma self-care, depressive symptoms, behavioral problems, emotional problems, and disregard of perceived asthma symptoms).

# MANAGING EXACERBATIONS OF ASTHMA

### MANAGING EXACERBATIONS OF ASTHMA—KEY POINTS

- Early treatment of asthma exacerbations is the best strategy for management. Important elements of early treatment include:
  - A written action plan to guide patient self-management of exacerbations at home, especially for patients with moderate-to-severe persistent asthma and any patient with a history of severe exacerbations
  - Recognition of early signs of worsening asthma
  - Appropriate intensification of therapy
  - Prompt communication between patient and clinician about any serious deterioration in symptoms or peak flow, decreased responsiveness to inhaled beta$_2$-agonists, or decreased duration of effect

- Management of asthma exacerbations includes:
  - Inhaled beta$_2$-agonist to provide prompt relief of airflow obstruction
  - Systemic corticosteroids, for moderate-to-severe exacerbations or for patients who fail to respond promptly and completely to an inhaled beta$_2$-agonist, to suppress and reverse airway inflammation
  - Oxygen to relieve hypoxemia for moderate-to-severe exacerbations
  - Monitoring response to therapy with serial measurements of lung function

Source: National Asthma Education and Prevention Program, *Expert Panel Report II: Guidelines for the Diagnosis and Management of Asthma*, National Heart, Lung, and Blood Institute, 1997.

## RISK FACTORS FOR DEATH FROM ASTHMA

- Past history of sudden severe exacerbations
- Prior intubation for asthma
- Prior admission for asthma to an intensive care unit
- Two or more hospitalizations for asthma in the past year
- Three or more emergency care visits for asthma in the past year
- Hospitalization or an emergency care visit for asthma within the past month
- Use of >2 canisters per month of inhaled short-acting beta$_2$-agonist
- Current use of systemic corticosteroids or recent withdrawal from systemic corticosteroids
- Difficulty perceiving airflow obstruction or its severity
- Comorbidity, as from cardiovascular diseases or chronic obstructive pulmonary disease
- Serious psychiatric disease or psychosocial problems
- Low socioeconomic status and urban residence
- Illicit drug use
- Sensitivity to *Alternaria*

Source: National Asthma Education and Prevention Program, *Expert Panel Report II: Guidelines for the Diagnosis and Management of Asthma*, National Heart, Lung, and Blood Institute, 1997.

## SPECIAL CONSIDERATIONS FOR INFANTS

- Assessment depends on physical examination rather than objective measurements. Use of accessory muscles, paradoxical breathing, cyanosis, and a respiratory rate >60 are key signs of serious distress.
- Objective measurements such as oxygen saturation of <91 percent also indicate serious distress.
- Response to beta$_2$-agonist therapy can be variable and may not be a reliable predictor of satisfactory outcome. However, because infants are at greater risk for respiratory failure, a *lack* of response noted by either physical examination or objective measurements should be an indication for hospitalization.
- Use of oral corticosteroids early in the episode is essential but should not substitute for careful assessment by a physician.
- Most acute wheezing episodes result from viral infections and may be accompanied by fever. Antibiotics are generally not required.

Source: National Asthma Education and Prevention Program, *Expert Panel Report II: Guidelines for the Diagnosis and Management of Asthma*, National Heart, Lung, and Blood Institute, 1997.

## MANAGEMENT OF ASTHMA EXACERBATIONS: HOME TREATMENT

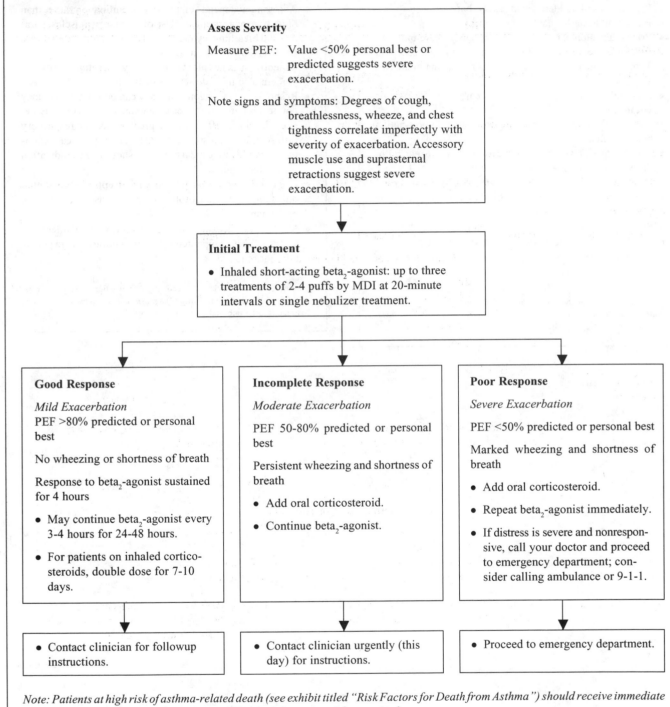

**Assess Severity**

Measure PEF:  Value <50% personal best or predicted suggests severe exacerbation.

Note signs and symptoms: Degrees of cough, breathlessness, wheeze, and chest tightness correlate imperfectly with severity of exacerbation. Accessory muscle use and suprasternal retractions suggest severe exacerbation.

**Initial Treatment**

- Inhaled short-acting beta$_2$-agonist: up to three treatments of 2-4 puffs by MDI at 20-minute intervals or single nebulizer treatment.

**Good Response**

*Mild Exacerbation*
PEF >80% predicted or personal best

No wheezing or shortness of breath

Response to beta$_2$-agonist sustained for 4 hours

- May continue beta$_2$-agonist every 3-4 hours for 24-48 hours.
- For patients on inhaled corticosteroids, double dose for 7-10 days.

**Incomplete Response**

*Moderate Exacerbation*

PEF 50-80% predicted or personal best

Persistent wheezing and shortness of breath

- Add oral corticosteroid.
- Continue beta$_2$-agonist.

**Poor Response**

*Severe Exacerbation*

PEF <50% predicted or personal best

Marked wheezing and shortness of breath

- Add oral corticosteroid.
- Repeat beta$_2$-agonist immediately.
- If distress is severe and nonresponsive, call your doctor and proceed to emergency department; consider calling ambulance or 9-1-1.

- Contact clinician for followup instructions.

- Contact clinician urgently (this day) for instructions.

- Proceed to emergency department.

*Note: Patients at high risk of asthma-related death (see exhibit titled "Risk Factors for Death from Asthma") should receive immediate clinical attention after initial treatment. Additional therapy may be required.*

Source: National Asthma Education and Prevention Program, *Expert Panel Report II: Guidelines for the Diagnosis and Management of Asthma*, National Heart, Lung, and Blood Institute, 1997.

## CLASSIFYING SEVERITY OF ASTHMA EXACERBATIONS

| | **Mild** | **Moderate** | **Severe** | **Respiratory Arrest Imminent** |
|---|---|---|---|---|
| **Symptoms** | | | | |
| Breathlessness | While walking | While talking (infant—softer, shorter cry; difficulty feeding) | While at rest (infant—stops feeding) | |
| | Can lie down | Prefers sitting | Sits upright | |
| Talks in | Sentences | Phrases | Words | |
| Alertness | May be agitated | Usually agitated | Usually agitated | Drowsy or confused |
| **Signs** | | | | |
| Respiratory rate | Increased | Increased | Often >30/min | |

Guide to rates of breathing in awake children:

| Age | Normal rate |
|---|---|
| <2 months | <60/minute |
| 2-12 months | <50/minute |
| 1-5 years | <40/minute |
| 6-8 years | <30/minute |

| | **Mild** | **Moderate** | **Severe** | **Respiratory Arrest Imminent** |
|---|---|---|---|---|
| Use of accessory muscles; suprasternal retractions | Usually not | Commonly | Usually | Paradoxical thoracoabdominal movement |
| Wheeze | Moderate, often only end expiratory | Loud; throughout exhalation | Usually loud; throughout inhalation and exhalation | Absence of wheeze |
| Pulse/minute | <100 | 100-120 | >120 | Bradycardia |

Guide to normal pulse rates in children:

| Age | Normal rate |
|---|---|
| 2-12 months | <160/minute |
| 1-2 years | <120/minute |
| 2-8 years | <110/minute |

| | **Mild** | **Moderate** | **Severe** | **Respiratory Arrest Imminent** |
|---|---|---|---|---|
| Pulsus paradoxus | Absent <10 mm Hg | May be present 10-25 mm Hg | Often present >25 mm Hg (adult) 20-40 mm Hg (child) | Absence suggests respiratory muscle fatigue |

*continues*

**Classifying Severity of Asthma Exacerbations** continued

| | Mild | Moderate | Severe | Respiratory Arrest Imminent |
|---|---|---|---|---|
| **Functional Assessment** | | | | |
| PEF<br>% predicted or<br>% personal best | >80% | Approx. 50-80% | <50% predicted or personal best or response lasts <2 hrs | |
| $PaO_2$ (on air)<br><br>and/or | Normal (test not usually necessary) | >60 mm Hg (test not usually necessary) | <60 mm Hg: possible cyanosis | |
| $PaCO_2$ | <42 mm Hg (test not usually necessary) | <42 mm Hg (test not usually necessary) | ≥42 mm Hg: possible respiratory failure (see text) | |
| $SaO_2$% (on air)<br>at sea level | >95%<br>(test not usually necessary) | 91-95% | <91% | |

Hypercapnia (hypoventilation) develops more readily in young children than in adults and adolescents.

Notes:
- The presence of several parameters, but not necessarily all, indicates the general classification of the exacerbation.
- Many of these parameters have not been systematically studied, so they serve only as general guides.

Source: National Asthma Education and Prevention Program, *Expert Panel Report II: Guidelines for the Diagnosis and Management of Asthma*, National Heart, Lung, and Blood Institute, 1997.

## DOSAGES OF DRUGS FOR ASTHMA EXACERBATIONS IN EMERGENCY MEDICAL CARE OR HOSPITAL

| Medications | Dosages | | Comments |
| --- | --- | --- | --- |
| | Adults | Children | |
| **Inhaled Short-Acting Beta$_2$-agonists** | | | |
| Albuterol | | | |
| Nebulizer solution (5 mg/mL) | 2.5-5 mg every 20 minutes for 3 doses, then 2.5-10 mg every 1-4 hours as needed, or 10-15 mg/hour continuously | 0.15 mg/kg (minimum dose 2.5 mg) every 20 minutes for 3 doses, then 0.15-0.3 mg/kg up to 10 mg every 1-4 hours as needed, or 0.5 mg/kg/hour by continuous nebulization | Only selective beta$_2$-agonists are recommended. For optimal delivery, dilute aerosols to minimum of 4 mL at gas flow of 6-8 L/min. |
| MDI (90 mcg/puff) | 4-8 puffs every 20 minutes up to 4 hours, then every 1-4 hours as needed | 4-8 puffs every 20 minutes for 3 doses, then every 1-4 hours as needed | As effective as nebulized therapy if patient is able to coordinate inhalation maneuver. Use spacer/holding chamber. |
| Bitolterol | | | |
| Nebulizer solution (2 mg/mL) | See albuterol dose | See albuterol dose; thought to be half as potent as albuterol on a mg basis | Has not been studied in severe asthma exacerbations. Do not mix with other drugs. |
| MDI (370 mcg/puff) | See albuterol dose | See albuterol dose | Has not been studied in severe asthma exacerbations. |
| Pirbuterol | | | |
| MDI (200 mcg/puff) | See albuterol dose | See albuterol dose; thought to be one-half as potent as albuterol on a mg basis. | Has not been studied in severe asthma exacerbations. |
| **Systemic (injected) Beta$_2$-agonists** | | | |
| Epinephrine 1:1000 (1 mg/mL) | 0.3-0.5 mg every 20 minutes for 3 doses sq | 0.01 mg/kg up to 0.3-0.5 mg every 20 minutes for 3 doses sq | No proven advantage of systemic therapy over aerosol. |
| Terbutaline (1 mg/mL) | 0.25 mg every 20 minutes for 3 doses sq | 0.01 mg/kg every 20 minutes for 3 doses, then every 2-6 hours as needed sq | No proven advantage of systemic therapy over aerosol. |
| **Anticholinergics** | | | |
| Ipratropium bromide Nebulizer solution (.25 mg/mL) | 0.5 mg every 30 minutes for 3 doses, then every 2-4 hours as needed | .25 mg every 20 minutes for 3 doses, then every 2 to 4 hours | May mix in same nebulizer with albuterol. Should not be used as first-line therapy; should be added to beta$_2$-agonist therapy. |
| MDI (18 mcg/puff) | 4-8 puffs as needed | 4-8 puffs as needed | Dose delivered from MDI is low and has not been studied in asthma exacerbations. |
| **Corticosteroids** | | | |
| Prednisone Methylprednisolone Prednisolone | 120-180 mg/day in 3 or 4 divided doses for 48 hours, then 60-80 mg/day until PEF reaches 70% of predicted or personal best | 1 mg/kg every 6 hours for 48 hours, then 1-2 mg/kg/day (maximum = 60 mg/day) in 2 divided doses until PEF 70% of predicted or personal best | For outpatient "burst" use 40-60 mg in single or 2 divided doses for adults (children—1-2 mg/kg/day, maximum 60 mg/day) for 3-10 days |

Note: No advantage has been found for higher dose corticosteroids in severe asthma exacerbations, nor is there any advantage for intravenous administration over oral therapy provided gastrointestinal transit time or absorption is not impaired. The usual regimen is to continue the frequent multiple dosing until the patient achieves an FEV$_1$ or PEF of 50 percent of predicted or personal best and then lower the dose to twice daily. This usually occurs within 48 hours. Therapy following a hospitalization or emergency department visit may last from 3 to 10 days. If patients are then started on inhaled corticosteroids, studies indicate there is no need to taper the systemic corticosteroid dose. If the followup systemic corticosteroid therapy is to be given once daily, one study indicates that it may be more clinically effective to give the dose in the afternoon at 3:00 p.m., with no increase in adrenal suppression.

Source: National Asthma Education and Prevention Program, *Expert Panel Report II: Guidelines for the Diagnosis and Management of Asthma*, National Heart, Lung, and Blood Institute, 1997.

## MANAGEMENT OF ASTHMA EXACERBATIONS: EMERGENCY DEPARTMENT AND HOSPITAL-BASED CARE

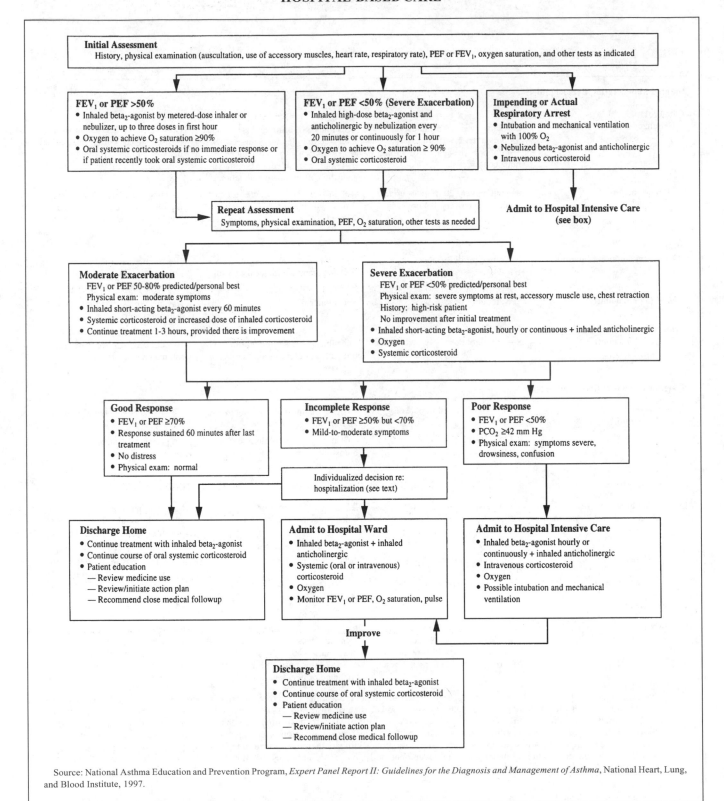

**Initial Assessment**
History, physical examination (auscultation, use of accessory muscles, heart rate, respiratory rate), PEF or $FEV_1$, oxygen saturation, and other tests as indicated

**$FEV_1$ or PEF >50%**
- Inhaled beta$_2$-agonist by metered-dose inhaler or nebulizer, up to three doses in first hour
- Oxygen to achieve $O_2$ saturation ≥90%
- Oral systemic corticosteroids if no immediate response or if patient recently took oral systemic corticosteroid

**$FEV_1$ or PEF <50% (Severe Exacerbation)**
- Inhaled high-dose beta$_2$-agonist and anticholinergic by nebulization every 20 minutes or continuously for 1 hour
- Oxygen to achieve $O_2$ saturation ≥ 90%
- Oral systemic corticosteroid

**Impending or Actual Respiratory Arrest**
- Intubation and mechanical ventilation with 100% $O_2$
- Nebulized beta$_2$-agonist and anticholinergic
- Intravenous corticosteroid

**Repeat Assessment**
Symptoms, physical examination, PEF, $O_2$ saturation, other tests as needed

**Admit to Hospital Intensive Care**
(see box)

**Moderate Exacerbation**
$FEV_1$ or PEF 50-80% predicted/personal best
Physical exam: moderate symptoms
- Inhaled short-acting beta$_2$-agonist every 60 minutes
- Systemic corticosteroid or increased dose of inhaled corticosteroid
- Continue treatment 1-3 hours, provided there is improvement

**Severe Exacerbation**
$FEV_1$ or PEF <50% predicted/personal best
Physical exam: severe symptoms at rest, accessory muscle use, chest retraction
History: high-risk patient
No improvement after initial treatment
- Inhaled short-acting beta$_2$-agonist, hourly or continuous + inhaled anticholinergic
- Oxygen
- Systemic corticosteroid

**Good Response**
- $FEV_1$ or PEF ≥70%
- Response sustained 60 minutes after last treatment
- No distress
- Physical exam: normal

**Incomplete Response**
- $FEV_1$ or PEF ≥50% but <70%
- Mild-to-moderate symptoms

**Poor Response**
- $FEV_1$ or PEF <50%
- $PCO_2$ ≥42 mm Hg
- Physical exam: symptoms severe, drowsiness, confusion

Individualized decision re: hospitalization (see text)

**Discharge Home**
- Continue treatment with inhaled beta$_2$-agonist
- Continue course of oral systemic corticosteroid
- Patient education
  — Review medicine use
  — Review/initiate action plan
  — Recommend close medical followup

**Admit to Hospital Ward**
- Inhaled beta$_2$-agonist + inhaled anticholinergic
- Systemic (oral or intravenous) corticosteroid
- Oxygen
- Monitor $FEV_1$ or PEF, $O_2$ saturation, pulse

**Admit to Hospital Intensive Care**
- Inhaled beta$_2$-agonist hourly or continuously + inhaled anticholinergic
- Intravenous corticosteroid
- Oxygen
- Possible intubation and mechanical ventilation

**Improve**

**Discharge Home**
- Continue treatment with inhaled beta$_2$-agonist
- Continue course of oral systemic corticosteroid
- Patient education
  — Review medicine use
  — Review/initiate action plan
  — Recommend close medical followup

Source: National Asthma Education and Prevention Program, *Expert Panel Report II: Guidelines for the Diagnosis and Management of Asthma*, National Heart, Lung, and Blood Institute, 1997.

**HOSPITAL DISCHARGE CHECKLIST FOR PATIENTS WITH ASTHMA EXACERBATIONS**

| Intervention | Dose/Timing | Education/Advice | MD/RN Initials |
|---|---|---|---|
| **Inhaled medications (MDI + spacer/holding chamber)** | Select agent, dose, and frequency (e.g., albuterol) | Teach purpose<br>Teach technique | |
| Beta$_2$-agonist | 2-6 puffs q 3-4 hr prn | Emphasize need for spacer/holding chamber | |
| Corticosteroids | Medium dose | Check patient technique | |
| **Oral medications** | Select agent, dose, and frequency (e.g., prednisone 20 mg bid for 3-10 days) | Teach purpose<br>Teach side effects | |
| **Peak flow meter** | Measure a.m. and p.m. PEF and record best of three tries each time | Teach purpose<br>Teach technique<br>Distribute peak flow diary | |
| **Followup visit** | Make appointment for followup care with primary clinician or asthma specialist | Advise patient (or caregiver) of date, time, and location of appointment within 7 days of hospital discharge | |
| **Action plan** | Before or at discharge | Instruct patient (or caregiver) on simple plan for actions to be taken when symptoms, signs, and PEF values suggest recurrent airflow obstruction | |

Source: National Asthma Education and Prevention Program, *Expert Panel Report II: Guidelines for the Diagnosis and Management of Asthma*, National Heart, Lung, and Blood Institute, 1997.

# PATIENT EDUCATION

## EDUCATION FOR A PARTNERSHIP IN ASTHMA CARE—KEY POINTS

- Patient education should begin at the time of diagnosis and be integrated into *every* step of clinical asthma care.

- It is essential that education be provided by *all* members of the health care team. The principal clinician should introduce the key educational messages and negotiate agreements with patients; these messages should be reinforced and expanded by all members of the health care team.

- Teach asthma self-management, tailoring the approach to the needs of each patient. Maintain a sensitivity to cultural beliefs and practices.

- Teach and reinforce at *every* opportunity:
  - Basic facts about asthma
  - Roles of medications
  - Skills: inhaler/spacer/holding chamber use, self-monitoring
  - Environmental control measures
  - When and how to take rescue actions
- Jointly develop treatment goals.
- To encourage an active partnership, provide all patients with a written daily self-management plan and an action plan for exacerbations. Action plans are especially important for patients with moderate-to-persistent asthma and patients with a history of severe exacerbations. Provide appropriate patients with a daily asthma diary.
- Encourage adherence by promoting open communication; individualizing, reviewing, and adjusting plans as needed; emphasizing goals and outcomes; and encouraging family involvement.

Source: National Asthma Education and Prevention Program, *Expert Panel Report II: Guidelines for the Diagnosis and Management of Asthma*, National Heart, Lung, and Blood Institute, 1997.

## ENCOURAGING ADHERENCE

An important part of patient education is encouraging adherence.

- **Use effective techniques to promote open communication.** Research suggests that certain clinician behaviors are associated with patient adherence and/or satisfaction with care. Use techniques such as making eye contact and praising effective management strategies.

- **Early in each visit, elicit the patient's concerns, perceptions, and unresolved questions about his or her asthma** (see exhibit titled "Delivery of Asthma Education by Clinicians during Patient Care Visits"). A question such as "What worries you most about your asthma?", which cannot be answered yes or no, encourages patients and families to voice issues, personal beliefs, or concerns they may be apprehensive about discussing or may not think are of interest to the clinician. These potential barriers to adherence can be dealt with only if they are identified. By asking about and discussing such concerns, clinicians build trust and a sense of partnership with the patient. Most nonadherence originates in personal beliefs or concerns about asthma that have not been discussed with the clinician. Until such fears and worries are identified and addressed, patients will not be able to adhere to the clinician's recommendations.

- **Assess the patient's and family's perceptions of the severity level of the disease.** Two questions may prove useful: "How severe do you think your asthma is?" and "How much danger do you believe you are in from your asthma?" When patients are identified who are overwhelmed by fear of death, put their fears in perspective by providing them with the results of objective assessments and expert opinion. A clearly written, detailed action plan that directs the patient how to respond to worsening asthma may be extremely helpful in reducing anxiety. Patients' perceptions about their disease severity and its threat to their well-being influence self-management behavior and use of the health care system.

- **Assess the patient's and family's level of social support.** Ask, "Who among your family or friends can you turn to for help if your asthma worsens?" Counsel patients to identify an asthma "partner" among their family or friends who is willing to be educated and provide support. Include at least one of these individuals in followup appointments with the patient so that he or she can hear what is expected of the patient in following the self-management and action plans.

- **Encourage or enlist family involvement.** Ask patients to identify ways their family members can help them follow the plans. Ask the patient to share the plans with family members, elicit their input, and agree on actions they can help with. It may be helpful for children and parents to discuss this with a clinician present.

- **Consider referral to a psychologist, social worker, psychiatrist, or other licensed professional when stress seems to unduly interfere with daily asthma management.** As with other chronic diseases, emotional and social stress may be a confounding factor for many patients struggling with asthma control. Although stress does not cause asthma, it can play a role in precipitating asthma exacerbations and can complicate an individual's attempt at self-management. Referral to a local support group may be useful.

- **Use methods to increase the chances that the patient will adhere to the written, daily self-management plan.** For instance, adherence to the self-management plan is enhanced when the plan is simplified as much as possible, when the number of medications and frequency of daily doses are minimized, when the medication doses and frequency fit into the patient's and family's daily routine, and when the plan considers the patient's ability to afford the medications. Because nonadherence is difficult for clinicians to detect, it is prudent to explore potential barriers to adherence with every patient by asking what concerns they have about medicines (e.g., safety) or other aspects of treatment.

Source: National Asthma Education and Prevention Program, *Expert Panel Report II: Guidelines for the Diagnosis and Management of Asthma*, National Heart, Lung, and Blood Institute, 1997.

# HOW TO INCREASE THE LIKELIHOOD OF COMPLIANCE

Patients cannot be expected to perform a task they never agreed to do or one that is mentioned only once to them. Thus, two essential clinician activities for successful patient education are:

1. **Asking the patient for a verbal, sometimes written, agreement** to take specific action(s). You will need to explain the recommended action(s) and the benefits the patient can expect from doing them.
2. **Following up** and reinforcing the patient for the actions during subsequent visits or phone calls.

**Other ways to increase compliance are:**

- **Develop an Asthma Action Plan with the patient** (see patient handout). Involve adolescents and school-age children in developing their plan, as appropriate. Minimize the number of medications and daily doses to the fewest clinically possible. Give parents additional copies of the plan to give to day care providers and schools.
- **Fit the daily medication regimen into the patient's and family's routine.** Explain the difference between long-term-control and quick-relief medicines and how to use them. Ask patients (and parents) when would be the easiest times for them to take their daily medicines.
- **Identify and address obstacles and concerns. Ask patients about problems they think they might have doing the recommended action(s).** Ask questions that start with "what" or "how" to identify the obstacles (e.g., "What are things that might make it hard for you to take the action each day?"). Discuss ways to address the problems or provide alternative actions.
- **Ask for agreement/plans to act.** Ask patients to summarize what recommended action(s) they plan to take, especially at the end of each visit.
- **Encourage or enlist family involvement.**
- **Follow up. At each visit, review the performance of the agreed-upon actions.** Praise appropriate actions and discuss how to improve other actions. Share evidence of the patient's improvement in lung function and symptoms. Remain encouraging when patients do not take the agreed-upon actions.
- **Assess the influence of the patient's cultural beliefs and practices that might affect asthma care.** Ask open-ended questions (e.g., "What will your friends and family think when you tell them you have asthma? What advice might they give to you?"). If harmless or potentially beneficial folk remedies are mentioned by the patients, consider incorporating them into the treatment plan.

## TEACH USE OF INHALER AND PEAK FLOW METER

Most patients use their inhalers incorrectly, and this skill deteriorates over time. Patients' poor technique results in less medication getting to the airways. The initial inhaler training can be done in minutes with the simple skills-training method described below. Note that different inhalers may require different inhalation techniques. The necessary reviews at each visit are quick and easy and can be done by other staff members in the office.

**Effective skills-training steps** for teaching inhaler techniques are as follows:

1. **Tell** the patient the steps and give written instructions. (For written instructions, see patient handouts.)
2. **Demonstrate** how to use the inhaler following each of these steps.
3. Ask the patient to **demonstrate** how to use the inhaler. Let the patient refer to the handout on the first training. Subsequently, use the handout as a checklist to assess the patient's technique.
4. **Tell** patients what they did right and what they need to improve. Have them demonstrate their technique again, if needed. Focus the patient on improving one or two key steps (e.g., timing of actuation and inhalation) if the patient made multiple errors.

**At each subsequent visit, perform the last two steps: patient demonstration and telling what they did right and what they need to improve.** Train patients to use their peak flow meter using the same four skills-training steps above and the patient handout in Part II, How To Use Your Peak Flow Meter.

## TIPS FOR REPLACING METERED-DOSE INHALERS

**The *only* reliable way to determine whether a metered-dose inhaler is empty is to count the number of puffs used and subtract the number from the total number of sprays in the canister.** Unfortunately, many patients believe they know when their inhalers are empty by floating the canister, spraying into the air, or tasting the medicine.

Clinicians and pharmacists can help patients determine the life of their long-term-control canisters by referring to the chart, How Often To Change Long-Term-Control Canisters, or by dividing the number of sprays per canister by the number of puffs prescribed per day. Determine the corresponding calendar date. Make an appointment before that date or make refills available after that date.

*continues*

**How To Increase the Likelihood of Compliance** continued

### How Often To Change Long-Term-Control Canisters

| # Sprays | 2 Sprays/Day | 4 Sprays/Day | 6 Sprays/Day | 8 Sprays/Day | 9 Sprays/Day | 12 Sprays/Day | 16 Sprays/Day |
|---|---|---|---|---|---|---|---|
| 60 | 30 days | 15 days | n/a | n/a | n/a | n/a | n/a |
| 100 | n/a | 25 days | 16 days | 12 days | n/a | n/a | n/a |
| 104 | n/a | 26 days | 17 days | 13 days | n/a | n/a | n/a |
| 112 | n/a | 28 days | 18 days | 14 days | n/a | n/a | n/a |
| 120 | 60 days | 30 days | 20 days | 15 days | n/a | n/a | n/a |
| 200 | n/a | 50 days | 33 days | 25 days | 22 days | 16 days | 12 days |
| 240 | n/a | 60 days | 40 days | 30 days | 26 days | 20 days | 15 days |

*If the medication is taken as prescribed, the canister should be discarded as indicated above. Otherwise, the remaining puffs may not contain sufficient medication.

Source: "Practical Guide for the Diagnosis and Management of Asthma" (Based on the *Expert Panel Report II: Guidelines for the Diagnosis and Management of Asthma*), NIH Publication No. 97-4053, National Heart, Lung, and Blood Institute, National Institutes of Health, October 1997.

## PATIENT EDUCATION FOR NON-CFC INHALERS

Clinicians need to be aware that metered-dose inhalers (MDIs) containing chlorofluorocarbons (CFCs) contribute to the depletion of stratospheric ozone. As a result of the consequent health hazards, CFCs have been internationally banned. Although a temporary medical exemption has been granted, MDIs with CFC propellants will eventually have to be replaced with alternative aerosol products, including MDIs with non-CFC propellants. Other non-CFC options include multidose dry powder inhalers and hand-held mininebulizers.

When first prescribing any of these new alternative products to patients accustomed to a CFC-containing MDI, the Expert Panel recommends that clinicians review with the patient the appropriate inhalation technique and care of the device to ensure proper use and optimum device performance. For alternative propellant MDIs, the patient may perceive differences in the aerosol delivery compared to their CFC-containing MDI. **The patient should be given the following messages about these differences:**

- **All FDA-approved alternative propellant inhalers will have been demonstrated to be comparably safe and effective as their usual CFC-propelled medication in clinical trials. However, individual differences in tolerability may be observed.**
- **Clinicians should familiarize patients with any differences in the care and use of non-CFC devices.**
- **The alternative propelled MDIs may taste different or feel different due to differences in the propellant and formulations. However, patients should be assured that these differences should not lead to important differences in their use of benefit.**

For alternate propellant MDIs that deliver a less forceful aerosol plume, patients may believe that this less forceful spray may not reach their lungs as effectively as their CFC product. Clinicians should reassure patients that medication delivery is assured by proper inhalation technique and that a less forceful spray does not equate with less efficacy. This is an opportunity to train patients in the use of non-CFC devices.

Source: National Asthma Education and Prevention Program, *Expert Panel Report II: Guidelines for the Diagnosis and Management of Asthma*, National Heart, Lung, and Blood Institute, 1997.

# Key Educational Messages for Patients

*Check off or document that the following key messages have been covered:*

## Basic Facts about Asthma

☐ The contrast between asthmatic and normal airways

☐ What happens to the airways in an asthma attack

## Roles of Medications

☐ How medications work

    – Long-term control: medications that prevent symptoms, often by reducing inflammation
    – Quick relief: short-acting bronchodilator relaxes muscles around airways

☐ Stress the importance of long-term-control medications and not to expect quick relief from them

## Skills

☐ Inhaler use (patient demonstrate)

☐ Spacer/holding chamber use

☐ Symptom monitoring, peak flow monitoring, and recognizing early signs of deterioration

## Environmental Control Measures

☐ Identifying and avoiding environmental precipitants or exposures

## When and How To Take Rescue Actions

☐ Responding to changes in asthma severity (daily self-management plan and action plan)

Source: National Asthma Education and Prevention Program, *Expert Panel Report II: Guidelines for the Diagnosis and Management of Asthma*, National Heart, Lung, and Blood Institute, 1997.

## DELIVERY OF ASTHMA EDUCATION BY CLINICIANS DURING PATIENT CARE VISITS

### RECOMMENDATIONS FOR INITIAL VISIT

| Assessment Questions | Information | Skills |
|---|---|---|
| *Focus on:*<br>• *Concerns*<br>• *Quality of life*<br>• *Expectations*<br>• *Goals of treatment* | *Teach in simple language:* | *Teach and demonstrate:* |
| "What worries you most about your asthma?"<br><br>"What do you want to accomplish at this visit?"<br><br>"What do you want to be able to do that you can't do now because of your asthma?"<br><br>"What do you expect from treatment?"<br><br>"What medicines have you tried?"<br><br>"What other questions do you have for me today?" | What is asthma?<br>A chronic lung disease. The airways are very sensitive. They become inflamed and narrow; breathing becomes difficult.<br><br>Asthma treatments: two types of medicines are needed:<br><br>• Long-term control: medications that prevent symptoms, often by reducing inflammation<br><br>• Quick relief: short-acting bronchodilator relaxes muscles around airways<br><br>Bring all medications to every appointment.<br><br>When to seek medical advice. Provide appropriate telephone number. | Inhaler and spacer/holding chamber use. Check performance.<br><br>Self-monitoring skills that are tied to an action plan:<br><br>• Recognize intensity and frequency of asthma symptoms<br><br>• Review the signs of deterioration and the need to reevaluate therapy:<br><br>  – Waking at night with asthma<br><br>  – Increased medication use<br><br>  – Decreased activity tolerance<br><br>Use of a simple, written self-management plan and action plan |

### RECOMMENDATIONS FOR FIRST FOLLOWUP VISIT (2 to 4 weeks or sooner as needed)

| Assessment Questions | Information | Skills |
|---|---|---|
| *Focus on:*<br>• *Concerns*<br>• *Quality of life*<br>• *Expectations*<br>• *Goals of treatment* | *Teach or review in simple language:* | *Teach or review and demonstrate:* |
| Ask relevant questions from previous visit and also ask:<br><br>"What medications are you taking?"<br><br>"How and when are you taking them?"<br><br>"What problems have you had using your medications?"<br><br>"Please show me how you use your inhaled medications." | Use of two types of medications. Remind patient to bring all medications and the peak flow meter to every appointment for review.<br><br>Self-evaluation of progress in asthma control using symptoms and peak flow as a guide. | Use of a daily self-management plan. Review and adjust as needed.<br><br>Use of an action plan. Review and adjust as needed.<br><br>Peak flow monitoring and daily diary recording.<br><br>Correct inhaler and spacer/holding chamber technique. |

*continues*

**Delivery of Asthma Education by Clinicians During Patient Care Visits** continued

### RECOMMENDATIONS FOR SECOND FOLLOWUP VISIT

| Assessment Questions | Information | Skills |
|---|---|---|
| *Focus on:* <br>• *Expectations of visit* <br>• *Goals of treatment* <br>• *Medications* <br>• *Quality of life* | *Teach or review in simple language:* | *Teach or review and demonstrate:* |
| Ask relevant questions from previous visits and also ask: <br><br>"Have you noticed anything in your home, work, or school that makes your asthma worse?" <br><br>"Describe for me how you know when to call your doctor or go to the hospital for asthma care." <br><br>"What questions do you have about the action plan?" "Can we make it easier?" <br><br>"Are your medications causing you any problems?" | Relevant environmental control/avoidance strategies. <br><br>• How to identify home, work, or school exposures that can cause or worsen asthma <br><br>• How to control house-dust mites, animal exposures if applicable <br><br>• How to avoid cigarette smoke (active and passive) <br><br>Review all medications. <br><br>Review and interpret from daily diary: <br><br>• Peak flow measures <br><br>• Symptom scores | Inhaler/spacer/holding chamber technique. <br><br>Peak flow monitoring technique. <br><br>Use of daily self-management plan. Review and adjust as needed. <br><br>Review use of action plan. Confirm that patient knows what to do if asthma gets worse. |

### RECOMMENDATIONS FOR ALL SUBSEQUENT VISITS

| Assessment Questions | Information | Skills |
|---|---|---|
| *Focus on:* <br>• *Expectations of visit* <br>• *Goals of treatment* <br>• *Medications* <br>• *Quality of life* | *Teach or review in simple language:* | *Teach or review and demonstrate:* |
| Ask relevant questions from previous visits and also ask: <br><br>"How have you tried to control things that make your asthma worse?" <br><br>"Please show me how you use your inhaled medication." | Review and reinforce all: <br>• Educational messages <br>• Environmental control strategies at home, work, or school <br>• Medications <br><br>Review and interpret from daily diary: <br>• Peak flow measures <br>• Symptom scores | Inhaler/spacer/holding chamber technique. <br><br>Peak flow monitoring technique. <br><br>Use of daily self-management plan. Review and adjust as needed. <br><br>Review use of action plan. Confirm that patient knows what to do if asthma gets worse. Periodically review and adjust written action plan. |

Source: National Asthma Education and Prevention Program, *Expert Panel Report II: Guidelines for the Diagnosis and Management of Asthma*, National Heart, Lung, and Blood Institute, 1997.

# Asthma Daily Self-Management Plan—Example 1

**ASTHMA SELF-MANAGEMENT PLAN FOR** _____

(Name)

## YOUR TREATMENT GOALS

☐ Be free from severe symptoms day and night, including sleeping through the night

☐ Have the best possible lung function

☐ Be able to participate fully in any activities of your choice

☐ Not miss work or school because of asthma symptoms

☐ Not need emergency visits or hospitalizations for asthma

☐ Use asthma medications to control asthma with as few side effects as possible

Add personal goals here: _____

_____

_____

## YOUR DAILY MEDICATIONS

| Daily Medication | How Much To Take | When To Take It |
|---|---|---|
| | | |
| | | |
| | | |
| | | |
| | | |

**RECORD DAILY SELF-MONITORING ACTIONS** in the asthma diary your doctor gives you.

**Peak flow:** At least every morning when you wake up, before taking your medication, measure your peak flow and record it in your diary. Bring these records to your next appointment with your doctor.

**Symptoms:** Note if you had asthma symptoms (shortness of breath, wheezing, chest tightness, or cough) and rate how severe they were during the day or night: mild, moderate, severe.

**Use of your quick-relief inhaler (bronchodilator):** Keep a record of the number of puffs you needed to use each day or night to control your symptoms.

**Actual use of daily medications**

**Activity restriction**

Source: National Asthma Education and Prevention Program, _Expert Panel Report II: Guidelines for the Diagnosis and Management of Asthma_, National Heart, Lung, and Blood Institute, 1997.

# Asthma Daily Self-Management Plan—Example 2

## Long-Term Self-Management Plan for Persistent Asthma

**Introduction:** This long-term plan provides four benefits to the clinician and patient, who complete it together during an early visit and review it periodically. The chart (1) reflects the step-up/step-down concept of pharmacotherapy; (2) enables patient and clinician to negotiate which medicines will be used and how often; (3) combines symptoms and/or peak flow monitoring as the basis for patient's adding or deleting medicines at home and self-adjusting doses; and (4) gives the patient a view of what the clinician recommends over the long-term—under what future circumstances the clinician intends that the regimen be increased or decreased.

**Directions:** The clinician writes the patient's medicines in the first column. Based on the symptoms and peak flow specified in the top row, the clinician then writes the doses and frequency of administration for each medication. (Some clinicians may prefer to print standard recommendations on the form to save time.)

| Medication | At the FIRST sign of a cold or exposure to known trigger | If cough or wheeze is present<br><br>or<br><br>peak flow is between 50 and 80% of personal best | If cough or wheeze worsen<br><br>or<br><br>peak flow is below 50% of personal best | As soon as cough and wheeze have stopped<br><br>or<br><br>peak flow is above 80% of personal best | When there is no cough or wheeze for 2 weeks, even with activity<br><br>or<br><br>peak flow is above 80% of personal best for 2 weeks | When there is no cough or wheeze for ___ months<br><br>or<br><br>peak flow is above 80% of personal best for ___ months | Before exercise or physical activity | For rapidly worsening asthma (severe exacerbation) |
|---|---|---|---|---|---|---|---|---|
|  |  |  |  |  |  |  |  |  |
|  |  |  |  |  |  |  |  |  |
|  |  |  |  |  |  |  |  |  |
|  |  |  |  |  |  |  |  |  |
| Times per day |  |  |  |  |  |  |  |  |
|  |  |  |  |  |  |  |  |  |

Source: National Asthma Education and Prevention Program, *Expert Panel Report II: Guidelines for the Diagnosis and Management of Asthma*, National Heart, Lung, and Blood Institute, 1997. Adapted from National Heart, Lung, and Blood Institute, *Asthma Management in Minority Children: Practical Insights for Clinicians, Researchers, and Public Health Planners*, National Institutes of Health publication number 95-3675, Bethesda, MD, 1995.

# Completed Sample—Long-Term Self-Management Plan for Persistent Asthma

Please note that the following long-term plan is included only as an example of how to fill out the plan. The treatment regimen itself does not correspond to recommendations made in the *Expert Panel Report II: Guidelines for the Diagnosis and Management of Asthma.*

| Medication | At the FIRST sign of a cold or exposure to known trigger | If cough or wheeze is present<br><br>or<br><br>peak flow is between 50 and 80% of personal best | If cough or wheeze worsen<br><br>or<br><br>peak flow is below 50% of personal best | As soon as cough and wheeze have stopped<br><br>or<br><br>peak flow is above 80% of personal best | When there is no cough or wheeze for 2 weeks, even with activity<br><br>or<br><br>peak flow is above 80% of personal best for 2 weeks | When there is no cough or wheeze for ___ months<br><br>or<br><br>peak flow is above 80% of personal best for ___ months | Before exercise or physical activity | For rapidly worsening asthma (severe exacerbation) |
|---|---|---|---|---|---|---|---|---|
| Short-acting beta$_2$-agonist | 2 puffs | 2 puffs | 2 puffs | 2 puffs | 0 | 0 | 2 puffs | 2-4 puffs |
| Nonsteroidal anti-inflammatory | 2 puffs | 2 puffs | 2 puffs | 2 puffs | 2 puffs | 2 puffs | 0 | 0 |
| Inhaled corticosteroid | 2 puffs | 4 puffs | 4 puffs | 2 puffs | 2 puffs | 0 | 0 | 0 |
| Antibiotic | | | | | | | | |
| TIMES PER DAY | 3 | 4 (every 4 hrs) | 4 (every 4 hrs) | 3 | 3 | 3 | 5-10 minutes before exercise | every 20 minutes for 3 doses* |
| Oral corticosteroid | 0 | 0 | 2 mg/kg/day × 2 days then 1 mg/kg/day × 3 days | 0 | 0 | 0 | 0 | 0 |

*If there is not a good response, seek emergency care immediately. If there is a good response, return to the third column.

Source: National Asthma Education and Prevention Program, *Expert Panel Report II: Guidelines for the Diagnosis and Management of Asthma*, National Heart, Lung, and Blood Institute, 1997. Adapted from National Heart, Lung, and Blood Institute, *Asthma Management in Minority Children: Practical Insights for Clinicians, Researchers, and Public Health Planners*, National Institutes of Health publication number 95-3675, Bethesda, MD, 1995.

# Asthma Action Plan—Example

Name _____ Date _____

It is important in managing asthma to keep track of your symptoms, medications, and peak expiratory flow (PEF). You can use the colors of a traffic light to help learn your asthma medications:

A. Green means Go—use preventive (anti-inflammatory) medicine
B. Yellow means Caution—use quick-relief (short-acting bronchodilator) medicine in addition to the preventive medicine.
C. Red means STOP!—get help from a doctor.

---

**a. Your GREEN ZONE is _____ 80% to 100% of your personal best. GO!**
Breathing is good with no cough, wheeze, or chest tightness during work, school, exercise, or play.
ACTION:
☐ Continue with medications listed in your daily treatment plan.

---

**b. Your YELLOW ZONE is _____ 50% to less than 80% of your personal best. CAUTION!**
Asthma symptoms are present (cough, wheeze, chest tightness).
Your peak flow number drops below _____ or you notice:
• Increased need for inhaled quick-relief medicine
• Increased asthma symptoms upon awakening
• Awakening at night with asthma symptoms
• _____.
ACTIONS:
☐ Take ____ puffs of your quick-relief (bronchodilator) medicine _____
   Repeat ____ times.
☐ Take ____ puffs of _____ (anti-inflammatory) _____ times/day.
☐ Begin/increase treatment with oral steroids:
   Take ____ mg of _____ every a.m. _____ p.m. _____.
☐ Call your doctor (phone) _____ or emergency room _____.

---

*continues*

**Asthma Action Plan** continued

---

**c. Your RED ZONE is _____ 50% or less of your best. DANGER!!**

Your peak flow number drops below _____, or you continue to get worse after increasing treatment according to the directions above.

ACTIONS:

☐ Take _____ puffs of your quick-relief (bronchodilator) medicine _____
   Repeat _____ times.

☐ Begin/increase treatment with oral steroids. Take _____ mg now.

☐ Call your doctor now (phone _____). If you cannot contact your doctor, go directly
   to the emergency room (phone _____).

Other important phone numbers for transportation _____.

---

**AT ANY TIME, CALL YOUR DOCTOR IF:**

☐ Asthma symptoms worsen while you are taking oral steroids, or

☐ Inhaled bronchodilator treatments are not lasting 4 hours, or

☐ Your peak flow number remains or falls below _____ in spite of following the plan.

Physician Signature _____    Patient/Family Member Signature _____

---

Source: National Asthma Education and Prevention Program, *Expert Panel Report II: Guidelines for the Diagnosis and Management of Asthma*, National Heart, Lung, and Blood Institute, 1997. Adapted from National Heart, Lung, and Blood Institute, *Asthma Management in Minority Children: Practical Insights for Clinicians, Researchers, and Public Health Planners*, National Institutes of Health publication number 95-3675, Bethesda, MD, 1995.

## 3. Clinical Pathway and Care Planning Forms

## Pediatric Ambulatory Asthma—4/5 Years and Older

| | First Visit | Second Visit | Third Visit | Fourth Visit | Fifth Visit |
|---|---|---|---|---|---|
| **Date** | | | | | |
| **Assessment** | Auscultation, RR, peak flow<br>Pulse oximetry if symptomatic | Auscultation, RR, peak flow | Auscultation, RR, peak flow<br>Weekly review of home diary | Auscultation, RR, peak flow<br>Weekly review of diary | Auscultation, RR, peak flow<br>Weekly review of diary |
| **Diagnostics and Treatment** | Office peak flow<br>Spirometry or pulmonary function testing<br>Chest X-ray<br>Labs: CBC, electrolytes<br>If symptomatic, treatment with beta-agonist with spacer device (or nebulizer) | Office peak flow<br>Beta-agonist treatment if peak flow in red zone | Office peak flow<br>Beta-agonist treatment if peak flow in red zone | Office peak flow<br>Beta-agonist treatment if peak flow in red zone | Office peak flow<br>Spirometry or pulmonary function testing |
| **Teaching and Counseling** | Correct use of MDI and meds<br>Introduce spacer device: InspirEase, AeroChamber, or Optihaler<br>Role of inhaled steroids in prevention of asthma | Reinforce correct MDI technique with spacer and/or without<br>Give flow meter and instructions for home monitoring<br>Teach warning signs<br>Instruct on trigger avoidance<br>Instruct on adverse effects of meds and what to watch for | Reinforce correct MDI technique<br>Set up temporary zones and discuss formulation of asthma treatment plan<br>Teach home monitoring of PEFR and meds<br>Instruct on trigger avoidance and environmental control | Reinforce correct MDI technique<br>Revise zones according to any new "personal best"<br>Discuss/revise home treatment plan: When to initiate oral steroids, proper use of MDIs with spacer for emergency relief, and, if necessary, nebulizer | Reinforce correct MDI technique<br>Make fine adjustments to home treatment plan |

*Note:* MDI, metered dose inhaler; NHLBI, National Heart, Lung, and Blood Institute.

*continues*

**Pediatric Ambulatory Asthma** continued

| | First Visit | Second Visit | Third Visit | Fourth Visit | Fifth Visit |
|---|---|---|---|---|---|
| Date | | | | | |
| Medications | Initiate inhaled steroids if not already in daily use<br>Inhaled beta-agonists<br>Mast cell stabilizer<br>Manage taper of oral steroid, if any | Inhaled steroids<br>Inhaled beta-agonists<br>Mast cell stabilizer<br>Taper oral steroids, if any | Stepwise approach to asthma meds (see NHLBI Guidelines) according to peak flow performance and symptoms | Continue stepwise approach<br>Step up (increase number of puffs)<br>Inhaled steroids for downward trend in home peak flow, trigger contacts, and other exacerbations | Step down and step up according to peak flow monitoring |
| Consults/Referrals/Additional Services | Smoking cessation for family members<br>Social worker<br>Visiting nurse for home assessment | Smoking cessation for family members<br>Establish communication with child's school health services | Smoking cessation for family members<br>Allergy clinic: Skin testing and evaluation for immunotherapy<br>Family calls provider if peak flow dips into low yellow zone or below | Smoking cessation for family members<br>Family calls provider if peak flow dips into low yellow zone or below | Smoking cessation for family members |
| Physiological Outcomes | Decreased dyspnea<br>Relief of symptoms with use of beta-agonists | Decreased dyspnea during activity<br>Improved daily peak flow | Minimal dyspnea<br>Peak flow in yellow and green zones | No symptoms<br>No limitation on physical activity<br>PEFR in high yellow and green zones | Full participation in home and school activities<br>PEFR in green zone |
| Medication Outcomes | Increased use of inhaled steroids for prevention<br>Minimal side effects of meds | Uses inhaled steroid daily for prevention of symptoms<br>Less frequent PRN use of beta-agonist<br>Minimal side effects of meds | Decreased need for PO steroids as inhaled steroid regimen is maintained<br>Less frequent PRN use of beta-agonist<br>Minimal side effects of meds | Daily inhaled steroid routine firmly established: Reducing number of puffs of inhaled steroid if PEFR stable<br>Infrequent need for PRN beta-agonist<br>Minimal side effects of meds | Uses minimal number of puffs of inhaled steroid to maintain personal best PEFR<br>Minimal need for inhaled beta-agonist<br>Minimal side effects of meds |

continues

**Pediatric Ambulatory Asthma** continued

| | First Visit | Second Visit | Third Visit | Fourth Visit | Fifth Visit |
|---|---|---|---|---|---|
| Date | | | | | |
| Educational Outcomes | Uses MDI properly, with/without spacer<br>Understands physiology of inflammation, bronchoconstriction, and hypersensitivity<br>Understands role of inhaled steroids in prevention of asthma exacerbations<br>Rinses mouth after inhaled steroid | Uses MDI properly with/without spacer<br>Uses home peak flow meter properly and knows how to maintain asthma peak flow diary<br>Knows personal warning signs | Uses MDI properly with/without spacer<br>Understands concept of zones: green, yellow, and red<br>Knows triggers to avoid | Uses MDI properly with/without spacer<br>Knows numerical ranges for own zones<br>Participates/understands formation of asthma treatment plan | Uses MDI properly with/without spacer<br>Can explain personal treatment plan:<br>Knows treatments to initiate at home and when it is necessary to come to office/ED for treatment |
| Psychosocial Outcomes | Child and family are comfortable using inhaled beta-agonist for the relief of symptoms and motivated to use inhaled steroid for prevention | Child and family are motivated to increase family management of asthma<br>Child is comfortable managing symptoms during school | Child and family gain increasing sense of control over asthma symptoms with ability to predict onset with peak flow monitoring | Child and family have greater sense of confidence in their ability to manage asthma at home | Child and family are confident of their skills to manage asthma at home and comfortable with asthma treatment plan<br>Able to comanage asthma effectively with provider and health care team |
| Comments | | | | | |
| Initials/Date | | | | | |

*Source:* Rufus S. Howe, *Clinical Pathways for Ambulatory Care Case Management*, Aspen Publishers, Inc., © 1996.

# Asthma Home Health Care Visit Plan

**First visit**, within one day of discharge from hospital (except weekends)

☐ Observation/physical assessment
☐ Initial home assessment and history for possible triggers
☐ Brief explanation of asthma
☐ Medication review and teaching including return demonstration of inhaler/spacer (Aerochamber)/ compressor-driven nebulizer (ProNeb)
☐ Review red zone signs and plan
☐ Discuss follow-up visits/when to call physician

**Second visit**

☐ Observation/physical assessment
☐ Complete asthma teaching, give home treatment plan based on age
☐ Introduce instructions on how to use a peak flow meter/introduce Asthma Peak Flow Diary
☐ Return demonstration of compressor-driven nebulizer/holding chamber/inhaler
☐ Completion of home assessment/instruct on how to avoid or eliminate trigger factors
☐ Verify physician follow-up/discuss plan for school setting

**Third visit**

☐ Observation/physical assessment
☐ Evaluation of understanding and compliance
☐ Review asthma peak flow meter use
☐ Review and reinforce physician's instructions
☐ Discharge instructions/review when to seek appropriate medication intervention

Source: Asthma Program Home Visit Protocol, developed for Principal Health Care by Pediatric Services of America, 3159 Campus Drive, Norcross, Georgia 30071. Used with permission.

# Skilled Nursing Facility Interdisciplinary Plan of Care—Asthma

| PROBLEM | GOALS | INTERVENTIONS | DISCIPLINES |
|---|---|---|---|
| **Asthma or Gas Exchange Impaired and/or Ineffective Breathing Pattern** | Rate ranging from ____ to _____ by/through: _____ | A. Asthma s/s <br> ___ Anxiety <br> ___ Dyspnea <br> ___ Respirations abnormal <br> ___ SOB <br> ___ Tightness in chest <br> ___ Wheezing | N |
| **R/T** | **And/or** | B. Causative factors | |
| ___ Asthma <br> ___ _____ <br> _____ | ___ Will report relief of chest tightness when asked by/through: _____ | ___ Make arrangements for allergy consult <br> Date: _____ <br> Recommendations for follow-through: _____ <br> _____ | S N |
| **Contributing Factors** | **And/or** | | |
| ___ Allergens <br> ___ Animal dander <br> ___ Dust <br> ___ Foods <br> ___ Mold <br> ___ Pollen <br> ___ Cold <br> ___ Exercise <br> ___ Irritants <br> ___ Air pollution <br> ___ Chemicals <br> ___ Smoke <br> ___ Unknown <br> ___ _____ <br> _____ | ___ Will have less than ___ episodes of asthma attacks by: _____ | ___ Elevate HOB ____ degrees | N NA |
| | | ___ Use ____ pillows to raise head | N NA |
| | **And/or** | ___ Provide ____ cc fluid/tray Offer additional fluid to ____ cc | D N NA |
| | ___ Will breathe without difficulty within ____ min of inhaler use by/through: _____ | ___ Notify/explain asthma to resident/family and encourage discussion of concerns | S N |
| **AEB** | **And/or** | ___ Respiration q ____ _____ | N |
| ___ Anxiety <br> Describe: _____ <br> _____ | ___ Will have no wheezing within ____ min of inhaler use by/through: _____ | ___ Incentive spirometry Frequency: _____ | N |
| ___ Dyspnea <br> ___ Respiratory range | | ___ Nebulizer treatments <br> ___ See physician order sheet, or <br> ___ Type/frequency:_____ | N |
| | **And/or** | | |

Resident's name: _____ Date: _____

*continues*

**Skilled Nursing Facility Interdisciplinary Plan of Care** continued

| PROBLEM | GOALS | INTERVENTIONS | DISCIPLINES |
|---|---|---|---|
| abnormal: _____ | ___ | ___ Adapt activity program to accommodate problem: | A |
|     Date(s): _____ | _____ | | |
| ___ SOB | _____ | _____ | |
| ___ Tightness in chest | _____ | _____ | |
| ___ Wheezing | _____ | | |
| ___ _____ | | Invite/escort to: _____ | |
| _____ | by/through: _____ | _____ | |
| ___ Will have respiration | ___ Assess/record/ report to MD prn | _____ | |
| | | ___ Resident education Check all that apply: | N S D A |
| | |   ___ Ask about air quality index before going outside | |
| | |   ___ Avoid causative factors | |
| | |   ___ Disease process | |
| | |   ___ Fluids (liquify secretions) | |
| | |   ___ Incentive spirometry | |
| | |   ___ Relaxation techniques | |
| | |   ___ Rest, need for | |
| | |   ___ _____ | |
| | | _____ | |
| | | ___ _____ | _ _ |
| | | _____ | _ _ |
| | | _____ | |
| | | _____ | |

# Part II

# Self-Management of Asthma: Patient Education

# About Asthma

**You cannot cure asthma, but you can control asthma.** People with asthma can have normal, active lives when they learn to control their asthma. They can work, play, and go to school. They can sleep well at night.

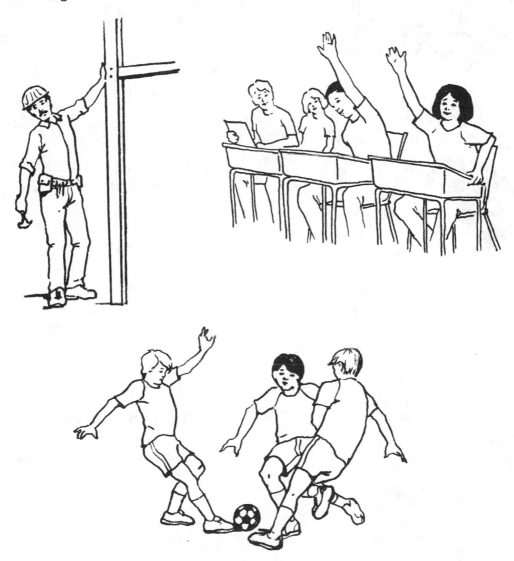

Asthma is not a cause for shame.

All over the world, many people have asthma.

*continues*

continued

## How to control your asthma and keep asthma attacks from starting:

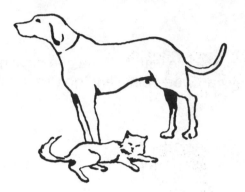

1. Stay away from things that start your asthma attacks.

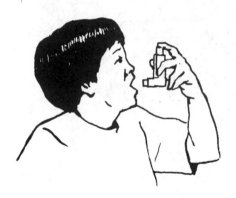

2. Take asthma medicines the way the doctor says to take them.

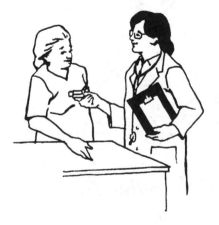

3. Go to the doctor two or three times a year for checkups. Go even when you feel fine and have no breathing problems.

*continues*

continued

**When you know there is asthma in the family, you may be able to keep your baby from getting asthma.**

- When you are pregnant, do not smoke.
- Keep tobacco smoke away from the baby and out of your home.
- Put a special dust-proof cover on the baby's mattress.
- Keep cats and other animals with fur out of your home.

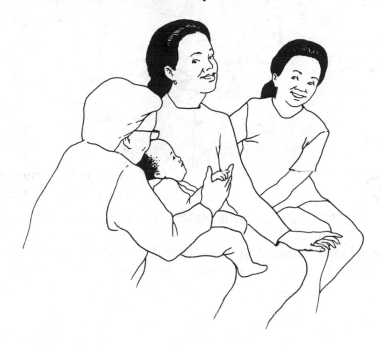

**People have asthma for many years.**

People with asthma can have trouble breathing. They have asthma attacks that come and go.

These are signs of an asthma episode.

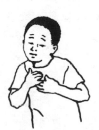   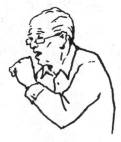   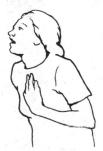

**Tight Chest          Cough          Wheeze**

*continues*

continued

Some asthma attacks are mild. Some asthma attacks get very serious. People can die from a bad asthma attack.

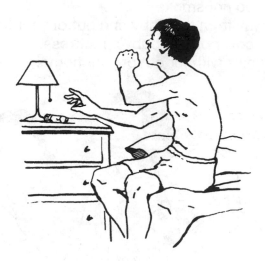

People with asthma may wake up at night because of coughing or trouble breathing.

**Asthma is a disease of the airways in the lungs.** You can get asthma at any age. You cannot catch asthma from other people. Many times, more than one person in the same family has asthma.

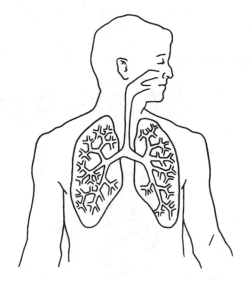

Airways carry air to the lungs. Airways get smaller and smaller like branches of a tree.

*continues*

continued

When asthma is under control, the airways are clear and air flows easily in and out.

Inside the airways, it looks like this.

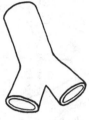

**When asthma is not under control, the sides of the airways in the lungs are always thick and swollen. An asthma attack can happen easily.**

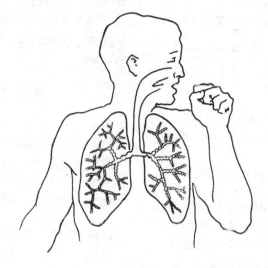

During an asthma attack, less air can get in and out of the lungs. People cough and wheeze. The chest feels tight.

During an asthma attack, it looks like this inside the airways of the lungs.

The sides of the airways get even more swollen.

The airways get squeezed.

The airways make mucus.

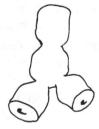

Source: "Global Initiative for Asthma, What You and Your Family Can Do about Asthma," National Heart, Lung, and Blood Institute, December 1995.

# What Is Asthma?

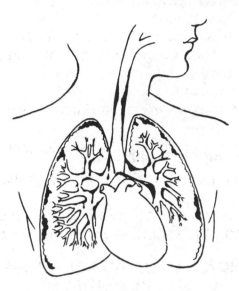

Asthma is a chronic lung disease that lasts a long time. It cannot be cured—only controlled.

- Airways are inflamed. That is, airway linings are swollen.
- Airways narrow and breathing becomes hard to do. This narrowing gets better (but not all the way in some patients), sometimes by itself, sometimes with treatment.
- Airways are super sensitive. They react to many things, such as cigarette smoke, pollen, or cold air. Coughing, wheezing, tight chest, difficult breathing, or an asthma episode may result. A more complete list of things that can cause some people's airways to react is given later (see "What Causes Asthma Episodes").

## WHAT ARE THE SYMPTOMS OF ASTHMA?

The main symptoms of asthma are:

- Shortness of breath
- Wheezing

- Tightness in the chest
- Cough lasting more than a week

Not all people with asthma wheeze. For some, coughing may be the only symptom of asthma. Coughing often occurs during the night or after exercise.

It's important to know that treatment can reverse asthma symptoms. And it's important to treat even mild symptoms of asthma so that you can keep the symptoms from getting worse.

## NORMAL BREATHING

When you breathe in, air is taken in through the nose and mouth. It goes down your windpipe, through your airways, and into the air sacs. When you breathe out, stale air leaves the lungs in the reverse order.

## WHAT HAPPENS DURING AN EPISODE OF ASTHMA?

Asthma affects the airways in your lungs. During an episode of asthma:

- The lining of the airways becomes swollen (inflamed)
- The airways produce a thick mucus
- The muscles around the airways tighten and make the airways narrower

These changes in the airways block the flow of air, making it hard to breathe.

You need to know the ways that asthma affects the airways so you can understand why it often takes more than one medicine to treat the disease. Very simply, some medicines

*continues*

continued

relax the airways, and others reduce (and even prevent) the swelling and mucus.

## WHAT CAUSES ASTHMA?

The basic cause of asthma is not yet known. What we do know is that asthma is not caused by emotional factors, such as a troubled parent-child relationship. In short, asthma is not "all in your head." It is instead a chronic lung disease.

## WHAT CAUSES ASTHMA EPISODES?

People with asthma have airways that are super sensitive to things that do not bother people who do not have asthma. These things are called triggers because when you are near or come in contact with them, they may start an asthma episode. Your airways may become swollen, produce too much mucus, and tighten up. Common triggers for asthma episodes include the following:

- Dander (or flakes) from the skin, hair, or feathers of all warm-blooded pets (including dogs, cats, birds, and small rodents)
- House-dust mites
- Cockroaches
- Pollens from grass and trees and mold
- Molds (indoor and outdoor)
- Cigarette smoke
- Wood smoke
- Scented products such as hair spray, cosmetics, and cleaning products
- Strong odors from fresh paint or cooking

- Automobile fumes
- Air pollution
- Infections in the upper airway, such as colds (a common trigger for both children and adults)
- Exercise
- Showing strong feelings (crying, laughing)
- Changes in weather and temperature

## IS THERE A CURE FOR ASTHMA?

Asthma cannot be cured, but it can be controlled. You should expect nothing less.

## HOW CAN ASTHMA EPISODES BE PREVENTED?

To prevent asthma episodes, you will have to work closely with your doctor to:

- Develop a medicine plan that keeps you from getting symptoms
- Plan ways to avoid or reduce contact with your triggers

## HOW ARE ASTHMA EPISODES CONTROLLED?

To control asthma episodes when they occur, you will have to work out a medicine plan with your doctor that includes:

- Treating symptoms early
- Doing the right things for any changes in symptoms
- Knowing when a doctor's help is needed and seeking help right away

*continues*

continued

---

## What Can a Patient with Asthma Expect from Treatment?

With proper treatment most people with asthma will be able to

- **Be active without having asthma symptoms. This includes participating in exercise and sports**

- **Sleep through the night without having asthma symptoms**

- **Prevent asthma episodes (attacks)**

- **Have the best possible peak flow number—lungs that work well**

- **Avoid side effects from asthma medicines**

**NOTES:**

Source: *Teach Your Patients about Asthma*, National Heart, Lung, and Blood Institute, October 1992.

# Common Questions and Answers about Asthma

**Q** Is asthma a major public health problem?

**A** Yes. Asthma affects over 100 million people worldwide and creates a burden in health care costs, lost productivity, and reduced participation in family life. Prevalence is increasing, most rapidly among children, especially where urbanization is taking place. This may be linked to factors including housing with reduced ventilation, exposure to indoor allergens (such as domestic dust mites in bedding, carpets, and stuffed furnishings, and animals with fur, especially cats), tobacco smoke, viral infections, air pollution, and chemical irritants.

**Q** Have solutions to the problem changed?

**A** Yes. Current information about causes as well as recently developed treatments to prevent attacks and strategies to manage asthma long term give us a new way to look at asthma.

**Q** What happens to a person who has asthma?

**A** A person with asthma has chronic inflammation of his or her airways, which can cause episodes (or attacks) of coughing, wheezing, chest tightness, or difficult breathing. Asthma symptoms come and go; they can last for a few moments or for days. Asthma attacks can be mild or severe and sometimes fatal. Medical care is usually required for severe attacks.

**Q** Who gets asthma?

**A** Asthma often occurs in families. It can occur at any age. It is not contagious. Asthma is a medical condition and not a cause for shame. Many Olympic athletes, famous leaders, and other celebrities have asthma. People can live successful lives with asthma.

**Q** What causes asthma?

**A** The exact cause is not yet known. It is clear that when people (especially infants) who have a family history of allergy are exposed to cigarette smoke or indoor allergens (such as domestic mites and cats), they have a strong likelihood of developing asthma. Some workers get it when exposed to certain inhaled chemicals.

**Q** Can asthma be prevented?

**A** Asthma episodes can be prevented, but more studies are needed to determine if development of the underlying disease can be prevented. Preventing exposure to environmental allergens and irritants may help prevent asthma.

**Q** Can asthma be cured?

**A** A cure has not yet been found. But it can be treated and controlled so that symptoms and attacks are prevented. Life with asthma can be mostly trouble free.

**Q** Will asthma change as a child gets older?

**A** Some children have fewer symptoms as they get older, and some have more, but this is not possible to predict. Asthma is a long-term condition. However, it is a condition that can be controlled.

**Q** How is asthma controlled?

**A** Because asthma is a chronic condition, it usually requires continuous medical care. Patients with moderate to severe asthma can take long-term medications (for example, anti-inflammatory agents)

*continues*

**Common Questions and Answers about Asthma** continued

daily to control the underlying inflammation and prevent symptoms and attacks. If symptoms occur, short-term medications (inhaled short-acting $beta_2$-agonists) are used to relieve them.

**Q**   Are medications the only way to control asthma?

**A**   No. It is important to avoid the stimuli that irritate and inflame the airways and make asthma worse. These are called asthma triggers. Each person must learn what triggers he or she should avoid.

**Q**   How does a person with asthma maintain control of his or her disease?

**A**   The person finds a knowledgeable physician who becomes his or her partner for long-term asthma management. Together they develop a management plan that specifies medications to take, triggers to avoid, and steps to follow if symptoms occur. Following the asthma management plan, and modifying it when necessary, may be a lifelong task.

**Q**   What can be expected from asthma management plans?

**A**   People who follow their asthma management plans can live active, productive lives and not often be bothered by asthma symptoms. Asthma management thus decreases the family, social, and economic burdens of the disease.

**Q**   How does asthma affect my community?

**A**   Your community may be spending too much on poorly controlled asthma. Individuals and families may have unnecessary financial and personal burdens from urgent care or hospitalizations. When people control their asthma, the whole community benefits from reduced asthma costs and increased productivity. Approximately 5 percent of the people in the world have asthma. If your community is undergoing urbanization, the proportion may be greater.

**Q**   How can I find out how large our asthma problem is locally?

**A**   Check local records on hospital and clinic visits, school attendance, and work attendance. Interview several families in your community about the kinds of problems asthma causes in their lives.

**Q**   Are the new treatments available in my community?

**A**   Probably. A variety of effective medications can be utilized, depending on available resources. Some new medications are expensive, but because they are effective, they prevent the need for most costly hospitalizations.

**Q**   Can we afford prevention and management programs?

**A**   Probably. In fact, because these programs are likely to save you money, you probably cannot afford to delay setting them up.

**Q**   Can I make a difference?

**A**   Yes! Physicians, nurses, educators, public health officials, and patients need to work together to manage and prevent asthma. This guide presents the most recent information about effective asthma management and prevention and suggests how this information can be adapted to reflect your local situation, resources, and cultural preferences. Any or all parts of this guide may be copied for use in your asthma program.

Source: "Asthma Management and Prevention," NIH Publication No. 96-3659A, U.S. Department of Health and Human Services, National Institutes of Health, December 1995.

# Datos sobre el asma

### ¿QUÉ ES EL ASMA?

El asma es una enfermedad crónica que inflama los pulmones y se caracteriza por problemas respiratorios recurrentes. Las personas que padecen de esta enfermedad tienen episodios agudos (algunos los llaman "ataques") cuando el paso de aire en las vías respiratorias se dificulta debido a la inflamación y la respiración se hace más difícil. Esos problemas son causados por una supersensibilidad de los conductos de aire pulmonares que reaccionan a ciertas "provocaciones" y consecuentemente se inflaman y se obstruyen.

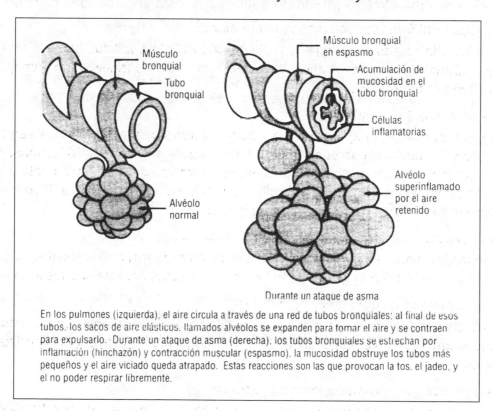

Durante un ataque de asma

En los pulmones (izquierda), el aire circula a través de una red de tubos bronquiales; al final de esos tubos, los sacos de aire elásticos, llamados alvéolos se expanden para tomar el aire y se contraen para expulsarlo. Durante un ataque de asma (derecha), los tubos bronquiales se estrechan por inflamación (hinchazón) y contracción muscular (espasmo), la mucosidad obstruye los tubos más pequeños y el aire viciado queda atrapado. Estas reacciones son las que provocan la tos, el jadeo, y el no poder respirar libremente.

De una persona a otra el asma varía en gran medida. Sus síntomas pueden ser leves, moderados o severos y hasta pueden poner en peligro la vida del individuo. Dichos episodios pueden ocurrir de vez en cuando o a menudo. Los síntomas del asma son una de las causas principales del tiempo perdido de los estudios, del trabajo y por trastornos del sueño. Sin embargo, con un tratamiento apropiado, estos síntomas casi siempre pueden ser controlados.

El asma es una enfermedad incurable, pero puede ser controlada con un tratamiento adecuado. Para aliviar los síntomas del asma, las personas afectadas pueden utilizar medicamentos recetados por sus médicos, para prevenir o aliviar sus síntomas, y pueden aprender algunas

*continúa*

continuación

formas de manejar sus episodios. También pueden aprender a identificar y evitar las cosas que provocan dichos episodios. Al educarse a sí mismos acerca de los medicamentos y de otras estrategias de control para el asma, la mayoría de las personas que padecen de esta enfermedad pueden controlarla y llevar una vida activa.

## ¿CUÁL ES LA CAUSA DEL ASMA?

No se conoce aún la causa básica de la anormalidad pulmonar en el asma. A través de investigaciones los científicos han logrado establecer que esta anormalidad pulmonar es un tipo de inflamación de las vías respiratorias que lleva a la contracción de los músculos respiratorios, a la producción de mucosidad y a la inflamación de las vías respiratorias. Las vías respiratorias se vuelven "espasmódicas" y responden excesivamente a los cambios del medio ambiente. Esto resulta en jadeos y tos. Algunos investigadores piensan que el jadeo y la tos pueden ser el resultado de una reacción anormal de los nervios sensores—que forman parte de la reacción inflamatoria.

Un episodio de asma puede ser desatado por una variedad de agentes:

- alergenos (sustancias a las que algunas personas son alérgicas), tales como el polen, algunos alimentos, el polvo, moho, plumas, o la caspa animal (pequeñas escamas de animales con pelo o plumas)
- irritantes en el aire, como el polvo, humo de tabaco, gases y olores
- infecciones de las vías respiratorias, como los resfríos, gripe, irritación de la garganta y bronquitis
- exceso de esfuerzo, como el subir escaleras corriendo o llevando cargas pesadas*
- estrés emocional, como el miedo excesivo o la excitación
- el estado del tiempo, como el aire muy frío, tiempo ventoso, o los cambios de tiempo repentinos
- medicamentos, tales como la aspirina o drogas similares y algunas drogas utilizadas para el tratamiento del glaucoma y la alta presión arterial

Cada persona con asma reacciona a un conjunto diferente de motivos. Un paso principal hacia aprender a controlar los ataques de asma es el de identificar los motivos que lo provocan en su caso particular.

Aunque algunos episodios pueden a veces ser ocasionados por fuertes emociones, es importante saber que *la causa* del asma *no* son los factores emocionales tales como una relación problemática entre padre e hijo. Algunas personas creen que el asma es algo que está "en la cabeza

*Sin embargo, se ha demostrado que el ejercicio moderado es de beneficio para muchas personas con asma. El ejercicio no debe ser descartado solamente porque uno padezca de asma.

*continúa*

continuación

de uno" y por lo tanto no es una enfermedad "real." Esto no es cierto. El asma es una enfermedad, no un mal psicosomático ni una señal de disturbio emocional.

## ¿QUIÉN CONTRAE ESTA ENFERMEDAD?

El asma ha sido diagnosticado en cerca de diez millones de personas estadounidenses; de ellas, tres millones son niños menores de 18 años de edad. El asma afecta casi al mismo número de hombres que de mujeres. La diferencia entre negros y blancos que sufren de asma es mínima— un 4.4 por ciento de americanos negros en comparación con 4 por ciento de americanos blancos.

El número de casos de asma está aumentando. Entre los años 1979 y 1987 el porcentaje de norteamericanos con asma aumentó en alrededor de un tercio, de 3 por ciento a 4 por ciento de la población. Este aumento se está produciendo en los grupos de todas las edades, razas y sexos.

El número de defunciones por asma ha aumentado de alrededor de 2,600 en 1979 a alrededor de 4,600 en 1988. La disparidad racial en las defunciones por asma es significativa y continúa en aumento: en 1979, las probabilidades de muerte por asma de los negros era el doble de la de los blancos, pero para 1987, la tasa de defunción por asma fue casi tres veces mayor entre los negros que entre los blancos. Sin embargo, la tasa de mortalidad por asma en los Estados Unidos es todavía una de las más bajas en el mundo, y es muy pequeña en comparación con el número de defunciones ocasionadas por las principales enfermedades mortales, tales como enfermedades del corazón, el cáncer y la apoplejía.

## ¿CÓMO SE DIAGNOSTICA EL ASMA?

Algunas veces es difícil diagnosticar el asma debido a que los síntomas son similares a los de otras enfermedades respiratorias, por ejemplo, enfisema, bronquitis e infecciones de las vías respiratorias inferiores. Por esta razón, es una enfermedad que está subdiagnosticada—muchas personas con la enfermedad no saben que la tienen—y por consiguiente, no es tratada. En algunos casos, el único síntoma es una tos crónica especialmente en horas de la noche. Otras veces, la tos y el jadeo ocurren sólo con el ejercicio. Algunas personas piensan que padecen de bronquitis recurrente, ya que, por lo general, las infecciones respiratorias se radican en el tórax en una persona con predisposición a esta enfermedad.

Para diagnosticar el asma y distinguirla de otros desórdenes pulmonares, los médicos confían en una combinación de la historia clínica, un examen físico exhaustivo y ciertas pruebas de laboratorio. Estas pruebas incluyen la espirometría (utilizando un instrumento que mide el air que entra y sale de los pulmones), el control del flujo máximo de aire (otra medida de la función pulmonar), las radiografías del tórax y en algunos casos análisis de sangre y pruebas de alergia.

*continúa*

continuación

## ¿EXISTE ALGÚN SÍNTOMA PREVIO A UN ATAQUE DE ASMA?

Por lo general, hay ciertas señales que aparecen unas horas o días antes del jadeo audible o de que el episodio llegue a desarrollarse plenamente. Estas señales varían muchísimo entre un individuo y otro. Algunas personas tienen una comezón en la barbilla o en la garganta o tienen la boca seca. Otras se pueden sentir muy cansadas o malhumoradas. Las señales de advertencia más comunes incluyen un leve jadeo o tos, dolor o sentimiento de opresión en el tórax, respiración corta e inquietud.

El reconocimiento de estas señales ayuda a las personas con asma a utilizar técnicas de autocontrol tan pronto como sea posible. Estas acciones preventivas pueden evitar un episodio severo.

## ¿QUÉ SUCEDE DURANTE UN ATAQUE DE ASMA?

Un episodio de asma es algo así como respirar profundamente aire muy frío en un día de invierno. La respiración se torna dificultosa y puede causar dolor, y puede haber tos. Al respirar, el aire puede producir un sonido jadeante o sibilante.

Estos problemas ocurren debido a que los conductos de aire de los pulmones se están estrechando; los músculos que rodean a los conductos se ponen tensos; la membrana interior de los conductos de aire se inflama y hace presión hacia adentro; y las membranas que recubren los conductos de aire segregan mucosidad en exceso que puede formar tapones que bloquean el paso del aire. La presión del aire al pasar a través de los conductos estrechos produce el sonido sibilante que es característico del asma.

Los ataques de asma van de un pequeño jadeo sibilante con tos o problemas de respiración, a ataques moderados que pueden ser controlados en el hogar, o a episodios severos que requieren ser tratados de emergencia por un médico. Algunos episodios son tan severos que pueden amenazar la vida del paciente y por lo tanto requieren atención médica inmediata.

## ¿QUÉ PUEDEN HACER LOS PADRES DE UN NIÑO CON ASMA PARA EVITAR O AMINORAR LA FRECUENCIA DE LOS EPISODIOS?

La clave para el control del asma es observar la condición del niño, tratar de prevenir los ataques y controlar un episodio tan pronto como comience.

Para prevenir los ataques, el niño afectado de asma debe evitar todas las situaciones que provocan el ataque y tomar medicamentos preventivos apropiados. Si el niño va a estar expuesto a una situación que ya sabe le provocará un ataque, tal como animales o ejercicios, puede tomar de antemano un medicamento para evitar el ataque.

*continúa*

continuación

Para observar la función pulmonar, el niño o sus padres pueden utilizar un aparato para medir el flujo máximo de aire. Este es un aparato pequeño, de poco costo, que sirve para medir la respiración, y que puede usarse en el hogar, en el trabajo o en la escuela. Debido a que la función pulmonar disminuye aún antes del comienzo de los síntomas de un ataque, el medidor asume la función de un signo de advertencia de un ataque. Al igual que un termómetro o un aparato para tomar la presión arterial, usado en forma apropiada puede ser una medida objetiva de la enfermedad. El uso de este aparato proporciona información para compartir con el médico, de manera que él y los padres puedan tomar decisiones acerca de la planificación del tratamiento a seguir.

A la primera señal de un ataque de asma, el niño debe parar y descansar, y tomar los medicamentos recetados para su enfermedad. Es importante hacer ésto tan pronto como se noten los primeros síntomas de aviso. De esta manera, un episodio serio, a menudo, puede prevenirse. Para los ataques de asma se usan diferentes tipos de medicamentos, de manera que es importante saber cómo utilizar cualquier medicina recetada y cuánto tiempo toma para que tenga efecto.

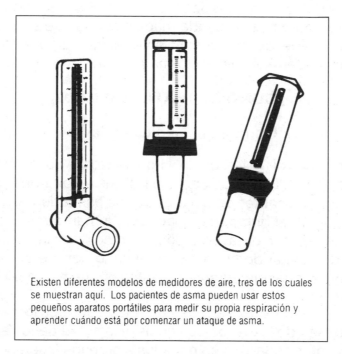

Existen diferentes modelos de medidores de aire, tres de los cuales se muestran aquí. Los pacientes de asma pueden usar estos pequeños aparatos portátiles para medir su propia respiración y aprender cuándo está por comenzar un ataque de asma.

Si los síntomas aún no mejoran, es importante consultar a un médico. Los niños asmáticos y sus padres deben saber cómo obtener asistencia médica rápida en caso de un episodio severo, y los niños deben tener algún compañero o amigo que pueda ayudarlos a llegar a una sala de emergencia o clínica. Las familias de niños asmáticos y sus médicos deben desarrollar un plan

*continúa*

continuación

de acción por escrito que sirva de guía para el tratamiento general del asma y para especificar el tratamiento cuando se desarrollen síntomas agudos. Dicho plan debe especificar qué medicamentos tomar, cuándo llamar al médico y cuándo ir a la sala de emergencia.

En resumen, a continuación figuran algunos alineamientos generales que pueden ayudar a prevenir o aminorar los episodios:

- Identificar y evitar los agentes provocadores de asma en su caso en particular. Sin embargo, si el ejercicio es uno de dichos agentes, considere el tomar medicamentos antes de hacer ejercicio.
- Tomar los medicamentos recetados a tiempo, de la manera correcta y en dosis correcta.
- Reconocer las señales tempranas de un ataque de asma.
- Leer el registro del medidor pulmonar para vigilar la función pulmonar.
- Tomar acción en cuanto se identifique un síntoma.
- Tener un plan personal para controlar los ataques elaborado conjuntamente con el médico.
- Tratar de tranquilizarse en caso de que esté por comenzar un ataque, saber qué hacer, y hacerlo.
- No espere demasiado para buscar ayuda médica cuando sea necesaria.
- Mantenerse saludable—descansar lo suficiente, alimentarse en forma apropiada, beber suficientes líquidos y hacer ejercicio en forma regular.

## ¿CÓMO SE TRATA EL ASMA?

### Control del medio ambiente

El primer paso hacia el control del asma a largo plazo es la eliminación de los factores desencadenantes. Por ejemplo, las infecciones de las vías respiratorias superiores, el humo del tabaco y los alergenos son causantes de los ataques de asma de muchos individuos. Tanto el fumar como el estar expuesto al humo del tabaco que fuman otras personas deben evitar las personas con asma. Pueden ser de ayuda algunas medidas simples, tales como reducir la exposición a los resfriados evitando el contacto cercano con personas que tienen resfríos y lavándose las manos con frecuencia durante la "estación de resfríos."

Los factores desencadenantes de asma más comunes son, por lo general, los de la alergia. Por lo menos el 90 por ciento de los niños con asma, y la mitad de los adultos con asma tienen alergias que agravan su enfermedad. Casi todos los alergenos (sustancias que causan alergia) que afectan al asma son inhalados. Estos factores incluyen partículas microscópicas de polen y moho exterior; y las polillas del polvo, caspa animal y moho interior. También pueden ser importantes los alergenos en los lugares de trabajo, por ejemplo, el polvo y los vapores provenientes de plásticos, granos, metales y madera.

*continúa*

continuación

El tomar medidas para evitar o eliminar algunos de estos alergenos puede mejorar muchísimo los síntomas del asma, aún en los casos de personas con asma severa. En general, las personas cuyos síntomas de asma no están bien controlados, que están expuestas a alergenos en el hogar o en el trabajo o que sospechan la presencia de factores alérgicos específicos deben solicitar al médico una evaluación del posible papel que tengan las alergias en su asma. De allí se podrán recomendar los cambios ambientales apropiados para mejorar el control del asma.

## Medicamentos

Los medicamentos son el fundamento del tratamiento del asma. Dado que el modelo de la enfermedad es diferente para cada persona, el tratamiento con un tipo específico de droga variará mucho dependiendo de la frecuencia, severidad y agentes desencadenantes particulares de los episodios de cada paciente. Por ejemplo, las personas con asma leve e intermitente, posiblemente tomen el medicamento sólo antes de exponerse a un agente desencadenante o cuando perciban los síntomas del ataque; mientras que aquellas con síntomas regulares pueden tomar el medicamento regularmente en dosis diarias para prevenir los episodios así como usar medicinas para síntomas específicos. Aquellas personas cuya enfermedad es severa y persistente pueden necesitar dos o más medicamentos diarios.

Aunque los laboratorios venden medicamentos para el asma bajo diferentes nombres, existen solamente unos pocos tipos principales.

## Agentes anti-inflamatorios

**Corticosteroides.** Estas son drogas antiasmáticas con creciente importancia que están dirigidas a reducir la reacción inflamatoria de las vías respiratorias. Se pueden obtener en píldoras y en forma de aerosol (para ser inhaladas). Debido a sus posibles efectos secundarios severos, el uso prolongado de esteroides por vía oral se reserva, por lo común, para casos severos de asma. Los esteroides inhalados, sin embargo, tienen menos efectos secundarios, son muy eficaces en la reducción de los síntomas y reactividad de las vías respiratorias, y parecen no ser dañinos para la mayoría de los pacientes.

**Drogas antialérgicas.** El cromolín sódico es la más conocida, junto con otras, tales como nedocromil y ketotifen, actualmente bajo pruebas clínicas. Las drogas antialérgicas son usadas para prevenir los episodios pero no surten efecto una vez comenzado el ataque. Estas drogas se usan mejor como medida de prevención diaria, pero tampoco son buenas para todos. Son más eficaces en las personas con asma leve o moderada.

## Broncodilatadores

**Broncodilatadores adrenérgicos (beta agonista).** Estas son medicinas que relajan los músculos de las vías respiratorias y las abren. Los broncodilatadores en aerosol (inhalados) son aspirados

*continúa*

continuación

a los pulmones usando un inhalador o nebulizador compresor. Los broncodilatadores adrenérgicos también pueden obtenerse en tabletas; sin embargo, su efecto es más lento que la del aerosol y tienen más reacciones secundarias, razón por la cual se prefiere la versión en aerosol. Los broncodilatadores se usan mejor cuando se necesitan—solos, si los síntomas son poco frecuentes, o como complemento de agentes anti-inflamatorios regulares.

*Advertencia:* Es peligroso depender sólo del uso de broncodilatadores inhalados cuando empieza un ataque. Los broncodilatadores sí dan una mejoría pasajera de los síntomas, pero no tienen efecto sobre la inflamación de los tejidos que realmente es la causa del episodio y por lo tanto no prestan una solución a largo plazo.

**La teofilina.** Este es otro tipo de broncodilatador. Se puede obtener en forma líquida, en cápsula o en tableta. Aunque la teofilina no es un broncodilatador tan fuerte como los medicamentos adrenérgicos, puede ser efectiva para algunas personas—por ejemplo, personas con asma nocturna—porque sus efectos tienden a ser más prolongados que los efectos de los broncodilatadores adrenérgicos. Los efectos secundarios son más comunes que con otros broncodilatadores y pueden incluir náusea, vómito y anormalidades del ritmo cardíaco.

**Los agentes anticolinérgicos.** Estas drogas, tales como la atropina, son las formas más antiguas de la terapia broncodilatadora para el asma. Sin embargo, actualmente se prefieren otros medicamentos porque tienen menos efectos secundarios y actúan más rápidamente para aliviar los síntomas del asma que los anticolinérgicos.

### Medicamentos de venta libre

Aunque estas medicinas pueden aliviar los síntomas temporalmente, a la larga son inadecuados, y pueden empeorar las cosas al ocultar una necesidad real de atención médica. Muchas personas con asma erróneamente tratan de automedicarse con esas medicinas, sólo para descubrir que cuando realmente necesitan ayuda, esas medicinas no son suficientes. Los únicos tratamientos efectivos para el asma son aquellos recetados, controlados y ajustados por un médico.

### Inmunoterapia

Para algunas personas alérgicas que no pueden controlar los síntomas del asma con cambios ambientales y medicamentos, la inmunoterapia (inyecciones de desensibilización alérgica) puede ser beneficiosa. Las alergias más exitosamente tratadas con inmunoterapia parecen ser las producidas por las polillas del polvo, el polen y los gatos.

*continúa*

continuación

## ¿RAZONABLEMENTE, QUÉ PUEDEN ESPERAR DEL TRATAMIENTO LAS PERSONAS CON ASMA?

Con un tratamiento apropiado, la mayoría de las personas con asma pueden esperar lograr:

- dormir toda la noche sin despertarse por la tos
- un tórax descongestionado por la mañana
- poder concurrir al trabajo o a la escuela con regularidad
- una actividad física total con un estilo de vida normal
- no tener que visitar la sala de emergencia ni hospitalizarse
- no sufrir efectos secundarios de los medicamentos

En el tratamiento del asma, los médicos buscan la supresión a largo plazo de la inflamación de las vías respiratorias que provocan los ataques de asma. Ya que en la actualidad el asma está reconocido como una enfermedad inflamatoria y no simplemente una contracción anormal de las vías respiratorias, el fin del tratamiento es el reducir la inflamación a largo plazo y abrir las vías respiratorias cuando se contraen.

## ¿PUEDE HACER EJERCICIOS LA PERSONA CON ASMA?

Por lo general, las personas con asma pueden y deben hacer ejercicios cuando se sienten bien. Puede ser necesario tener un cuidado especial cuando el aire es frío o durante las estaciones del polen. Siempre es mejor comenzar despacio e ir aumentando el ejercicio poco a poco, y es esencial consultar con el médico antes de comenzar cualquier tipo de ejercicio regular. A menudo, usar un broncodilatador adrenérgico inhalado antes de los ejercicios puede evitar los síntomas inducidos por el ejercicio y permitir que la persona sea totalmente activa. Las personas asmáticas no deben creer que necesitan limitar sus actividades físicas simplemente porque tienen la enfermedad; después de todo, algunos atletas olímpicos tienen asma severa. A las personas no se les debe restringir las actividades físicas simplemente porque tienen asma.

## ¿ESTÁN LOS CIENTÍFICOS HACIENDO INVESTIGACIONES QUE PODRÍAN AYUDAR A LAS PERSONAS CON ASMA?

Los investigadores están trabajando en varios frentes para contestar algunas de las muchas preguntas que están sin contestar con respecto al asma. En los Institutos Nacionales de Salud, la investigación sobre el asma es llevada a cabo y apoyada por dos unidades, el Instituto Nacional del Corazón, los Pulmones y la Sangre (NHLBI) y el Instituto Nacional de Alergia y Enfermedades Infecciosas. Los proyectos patrocinados por dichas agencias están encaminados a identificar las anormalidades básicas que causan el asma, al desarrollo de mejores drogas para los tratamientos y mejores medidas de emergencia, y a educar a las personas con asma para que se ayuden a sí mismas.

*continúa*

continuación

Investigaciones patrocinadas por el NHLBI han establecido que los progamas educativos pueden reducir muchísimo las hospitalizaciones e incapacidades por asma. En esos programas, los pacientes son capacitados en técnicas de autocontrol del asma mientras están bajo supervisión médica. Basado en ésta y otros conocimientos derivados de las investigaciones, el NHLBI comenzó, en marzo de 1989, el Programa Nacional de Educación para el Asma. Este esfuerzo nacional está dirigido a aumentar los conocimientos del público sobre el asma como una enfermedad crónica seria, a asegurar su diagnóstico apropiado y a permitir un control efectivo de la enfermedad promoviendo una alianza entre pacientes, médicos y otros profesionales del cuidado de la salud por medio de tratamientos modernos y de programas educacionales.

**Para obtener más información sobre el asma, diríjase a**

National Asthma Education Program
Information Center
P.O. Box 30105
Bethesda, MD 20824-0105
(301) 951-3260

Pida la lista de literatura y recursos para el asma, donde encontrará muchas fuentes de información más específica sobre varios aspectos de la enfermedad.

**NOTAS:**

Source: "El Asma," National Heart, Lung, and Blood Institute.

# Controlling Your Asthma

## HOW TO TAKE CARE OF YOUR ASTHMA

1. **Work with your doctor and see him or her at least every 6 months.**
   *See:*
   "How To Work with Your Doctor" (on this page)

2. **Take your asthma medicines exactly as your doctor tells you.**

3. **Watch for signs that your asthma is getting worse and act quickly.**

4. **Stay away from or control things that make your asthma worse.**

## HOW TO WORK WITH YOUR DOCTOR

- **Agree on clear treatment goals with your doctor.** Your goal is to be able to say "no" to all the questions in the box titled, "Is Your Asthma under Control?"
- **Agree on what things you need to do. Then do them.**
   - Ask questions until you feel you know what your doctor wants you to do, when you should do it, and why. Tell your doctor if you think you will have trouble doing what is asked. You can work together to find a treatment plan that is right for you.
   - Write down the things you are supposed to do before you leave the doctor's office, or soon after.
   - Put up reminders to yourself to take your medicine on time. Put these notes in places where you will see them.

- **See your doctor at least every 6 months to check your asthma and review your treatment.** Call for an appointment if you need one.

## PREPARE A DAY OR TWO BEFORE EACH DOCTOR'S VISIT:

- **Answer the questions in "Is Your Asthma under Control?".** Talk to your doctor about your answers. Also, talk about any changes in your home or work that may have made your asthma worse.
- **Write down questions and concerns to discuss with your doctor.** Include ALL of your concerns, even those you think are not a big deal.
- **Bring your medicines and written action plan to each visit.** If you use a peak flow meter, bring it to each visit.

> **"The doctor would ask me at each visit how little Jimmy's asthma was. I always forgot to mention some symptoms or other problems. Now it's different. Before we visit the doctor, I write down when Jimmy had symptoms in the past 2 weeks. I also write down all the questions I have. Now when I leave the doctor's office, I feel happy that I got all my issues addressed."**
>
> *Deborah, mother of a child with asthma*

Source: "Controlling Your Asthma," NIH Publication No. 97-4053, U.S. Department of Health and Human Services, National Heart, Lung, and Blood Institute, National Institutes of Health, October 1997.

# Is Your Asthma under Control?

Answer these questions by checking "yes" or "no." Do this just before each doctor's visit.

**In the past 2 weeks:**

1. Have you coughed, wheezed, felt short of breath, or had chest tightness?

   - During the day? ___ yes    ___ no
   - At night, causing you to wake up? ___ yes    ___ no
   - During or soon after exercise? ___ yes    ___ no

2. Have you needed more "quick-relief" medicine than usual? ___ yes    ___ no

3. Has your asthma kept you from doing *anything* you wanted to do? ___ yes    ___ no

   If yes, what was it?

   _____

   _____

4. Have your asthma medicines caused you any problems, like
   shakiness, sore throat, or upset stomach? ___ yes    ___ no

**In the past few months:**

5. Have you missed school or work because of your asthma? ___ yes    ___ no

6. Have you gone to the emergency room or hospital because of
   your asthma? ___ yes    ___ no

**What Your Answers Mean**

**All "no" answers?—Your asthma is under control.**
Read this guide to help you keep your asthma under control.

**One or more "yes" answers?—Something needs to be done.**
Talk to your doctor to find out how to get your asthma under control.

Source: "Controlling Your Asthma," NIH Publication No. 97-4053, U.S. Department of Health and Human Services, National Heart, Lung, and Blood Institute, National Institutes of Health, October 1997.

# ¿Está su asma bajo control?

Conteste estas preguntas con un "sí" o un "no." Haga esto antes de cada visita al médico.

**En las últimas 2 semanas:**

1. ¿Ha tosido, ha tenido silbidos (pitillo, ronquera o hervor de pecho), dificultad en respirar o ha sentido presión, tirantez o apretazón en el pecho?

   - ¿Durante el día?                                          ___ sí ___ no
   - ¿En la noche y lo hizo despertar?                         ___ sí ___ no
   - ¿Durante o después de hacer ejercicio?                    ___ sí ___ no

2. ¿Ha necesitado usar más de su medicina "para el alivio rápido" de la que acostumbra tomar?                                ___ sí ___ no

3. ¿Le ha impedido el asma hacer *algo* que quería hacer?     ___ sí ___ no

   Si la respuesta es "sí", ¿qué fué?

4. ¿Le han causado algún problema las medicinas que toma para el asma, tales como tembladera, dolor de garganta o malestar en el estómago?                                              ___ sí ___ no

**En los últimos meses:**

5. ¿Ha faltado a la escuela o al trabajo por causa del asma?   ___ sí ___ no

6. ¿Ha ido a la sala de emergencia o al hospital por causa del asma?   ___ sí ___ no

**Lo que significan sus respuestas**

**¿Contestó "no" a todas las preguntas?—Su asma está bajo control.** Lea esta guía para que le ayude a mantener su asma bajo control.

**¿Contestó "sí" a una o más preguntas?—Tiene que hacer algo.** Lea esta guía y háblele a su médico para averiguar cómo poner su asma bajo control.

Source: *Facts About Controlling Asthma,* National Asthma Education and Prevention Program, National Heart, Lung, and Blood Institute, NIH Publication No. 97-2339.

# Cómo controlar las cosas que empeoran su asma

Usted puede ayudar a prevenir los ataques de asma si evita ciertas cosas que empeoran la enfermedad. En esta guía se sugieren muchas maneras de hacerlo.

Será necesario que usted se fije qué cosas empeoran *su* asma. Algunas cosas que empeoran el asma de algunas personas no son un problema para otras. Usted no tiene que hacer todo lo que se indica en esta guía.

Mire las cosas que aparecen a continuación en letra más oscura. Ponga una marca al lado de las que sabe que empeoran su asma. Pídale a su médico que le ayude a encontrar qué otras cosas lo empeoran. Luego decida con su médico, qué medidas tomar. Comience con las cosas en su *dormitorio* que empeoran su asma. Trate primero algo que sea fácil de cambiar.

### Humo de tabaco

- Si fuma, pídale a su médico que le indique distintas maneras de dejar de hacerlo. Pídale a sus familiares que también dejen de fumar.
- No permita que se fume en su casa o a su alrededor.
- Asegúrese de que nadie fume en una guardería de niños.

### Los ácaros del polvo

Muchas personas con asma son alérgicas a los ácaros del polvo. Los ácaros son animales pequeñísimos que no se pueden ver y viven en telas o alfombras.

**Cosas que le ayudarán más:**

- Ponga su colchón dentro de una funda especial a prueba de polvo.
- Ponga su almohada dentro de una funda especial a prueba de polvo o lave la almohada todas las semanas con agua caliente. Se necesita agua a una temperatura más alta de los 130°F para matar los ácaros.
- Lave todas las semanas, con agua caliente, las sábanas y frazadas de su cama.

**Otras cosas que le pueden ayudar:**

- Baje la humedad del interior de su casa, a menos del 50 por ciento. Los deshumidificadores o los acondicionadores de aire centrales pueden hacer esto.
- Trate de no dormir, ni acostarse, en muebles o almohadones forrados de tela.
- Si puede, saque las alfombras de su dormitorio y las que están sobre piso de concreto.
- Saque de la cama los juguetes de felpa o peluche o lávelos todas las semanas con agua caliente.

*continúa*

continuación

## Caspa de los animales

Algunas personas son alérgicas a las escamas (o caspa) de la piel de algunos animals o a la saliva seca de los animales peludos o con plumas, como por ejemplo el gato.

**Lo mejor que puede hacer:**

- Mantenga a los animales peludos o con plumas fuera de la casa.

**Si no puede dejar a los animales fuera de la casa, entonces:**

- Deje al animal fuera de su dormitorio y mantenga la puerta siempre cerrada.
- Cubra las salidas de aire de su dormitorio con tela gruesa para filtrar el aire.
- Saque de su casa las alfombras y los muebles forrados de tela. Si eso no es posible, mantenga al animal fuera de las habitaciones con alfombras y muebles forrados de tela.

## Cucarachas

Muchas personas con asma son alérgicas a los excrementos secos y restos de cucarachas.

- Mantenga todo alimento fuera de su dormitorio.
- Guarde siempre los alimentos y mantenga la basura en recipientes cerrados (nunca deje alimentos afuera).
- Use cebo con veneno, polvos, gelatinas o gastas (por ejemplo, ácido bórico). También puede usar trampas.
- Si usa un "spray" (rociador) para matar cucarachas, permanezca fuera de la habitación hasta que se vaya el olor.

## Limpieza con aspiradora

- Si puede, trate de conseguir que alguien pase la aspiradora por usted, una o dos veces por semana. Quédese fuera de las habitaciones mientras están pasando la aspiradora o acaben de pasarla.
- Si usted pasa la aspiradora, use una mascarilla contra el polvo (se encuentran en las ferreterías), una bolsa para la aspiradora, de doble capa o con microfiltro, o una aspiradora con un tipo de filtro llamado HEPA.

## Moho (hongos) en el interior de la casa

- Repare los grifos (llaves o chorros), cañerías u otras fuentes de agua que gotean.
- Limpie las superficies que tengan moho con un limpiador que tenga lejía ("bleach").

*continúa*

continuación

## El polen y el moho fuera de la casa

Qué hacer durante la estación de las alergias (cuando la cantidad de polen y esporas de moho es alta):

- Trate de mantener las ventanas cerradas.
- Si puede, quédese dentro de la casa con las ventanas cerradas durante las horas del mediodía y la tarde. Es durante esas horas que aumenta la cantidad de polen y de algunas esporas del moho.
- Pregunte a su médico si necesita tomar o aumentar la cantidad de medicina anti-inflamatoria antes de que comience el tiempo o la estación en que aparecen sus alergias.

## Humo, olores fuertes y rociadores ("sprays")

- De ser posible, no use cocina de leña, estufas de querosén ni chimenea.
- Trate de mantenerse alejado de los olores fuertes y rociadores, como perfume, talco, aerosoles para el cabello y pinturas.

## Ejercicio, deportes, trabajo o juegos

- Usted debe poder mantenerse activo y sin síntomas. Pero vea a su médico si aparecen los síntomas de asma cuando hace ejercicio.
- Pregunte a su médico si es aconsejable tomar la medicina antes de hacer ejercicio para prevenir los síntomas.
- "Caliente" su cuerpo por unos 6 a 10 minutos, antes de hacer ejercicio.
- Trate de no trabajar o jugar mucho al aire libre, cuando la contaminación del air o los niveles de polen (si es alérgico al polen) son altos.

## Otras cosas que pueden empeorar el asma

- Influenza (gripe): Hágase aplicar la vacuna contra la influenza.
- No coma alimentos que contiennen sulfitos ("sulfites"): No beba cerveza ni vino y no coma camarones, frutas secas ni papas preparadas, si le producen síntomas de asma.
- Aire frío: Cúbrase la nariz y la boca con una bufanda en los días fríos y con vientos.
- Otras medicinas: Informe a su médico sobre todas las medicinas que pueda estar tomando, inclusive remedios caseros, medicinas compradas en otro país o regaladas por un amigo o familiar, medicinas para el resfrío, aspirina y aún gotas para los ojos.

Source: *Facts About Controlling Asthma*, National Asthma Education and Prevention Program, National Heart, Lung, and Blood Institute, NIH Publication No. 97-2339.

# About Peak Flow Meters

**A peak flow meter can be used at a clinic or at home to measure how well a person is breathing.**

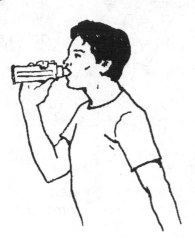

- It helps the doctor decide if someone has asthma
- It helps to see how bad an asthma attack is
- It helps the doctor see how well asthma is controlled over time

If you use a peak flow meter every day at home, you can find breathing problems even before you start to wheeze or cough. Then you know when more asthma medicine is needed.

There are many kinds of peak flow meters.

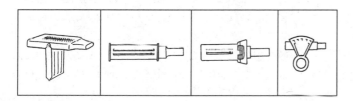

**How to use a peak flow meter**

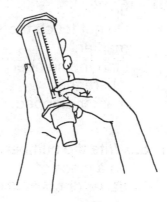

1. Slide the little marker down as far as it will go. This sets the meter to zero.

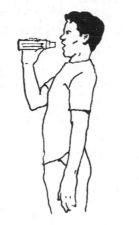

2. Stand up.
   Take a big breath with your mouth open.
   Hold the meter in one hand.
   Keep your fingers away from the numbers.

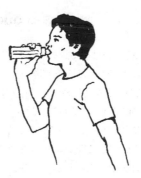

3. Quickly close your lips firmly around the tube.
   Do not put your tongue in the hole.
   Blow one time as fast and hard as you can.

*continues*

continued

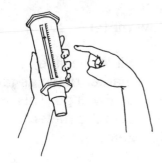

4. The marker will
   go up and stay
   up.
   Do not touch the
   marker.
   Find the number
   where the
   marker stopped.

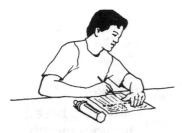

5. Write the number
   on a piece of
   paper or on a
   chart.

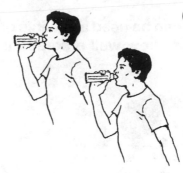

6. Blow two more
   times.
   Push the button
   down each time.
   Write the number
   down each time.

**NOTES:**

Source: "Global Initiative for Asthma, What You and Your Family Can Do about Asthma," National Heart, Lung, and Blood Institute, December 1995.

# How To Use Your Peak Flow Meter

## INTRODUCTION

A peak flow meter is a device that measures how well air moves out of your lungs. During an asthma episode the airways of the lungs begin to narrow slowly. The peak flow meter will tell you if there is narrowing in the airways days—even hours—before you have any symptoms of asthma.

By taking your medicine(s) early (before symptoms), you may be able to stop the episode quickly and avoid a severe episode of asthma. Peak flow meters are used to check your asthma the way that blood pressure cuffs are used to check high blood pressure.

The peak flow meter can also be used to help you and your doctor:

- learn what makes your asthma worse
- decide if your medicine plan is working well
- decide when to add or stop medicine
- decide when to seek emergency care

A peak flow meter is most helpful for patients who must take asthma medicine every day. Patients age 5 and older are able to use a peak flow meter. Ask your doctor or nurse to show you how to use a peak flow meter.

## HOW TO USE YOUR PEAK FLOW METER

- Do the following five steps with your peak flow meter:
  1. Put the indicator at the bottom of the numbered scale.
  2. Stand up.
  3. Take a deep breath.
  4. Place the meter in your mouth and close your lips around the mouthpiece. Do not put your tongue inside the hole.
  5. Blow out as hard and fast as you can.
- Write down the number you get.
- Repeat steps 1 through 5 two more times and write down the numbers you get.
- Write down in "My Asthma Symptoms and Peak Flow Diary" the highest of the three numbers achieved.

## FIND YOUR PERSONAL BEST PEAK FLOW NUMBER

Your **personal best** peak flow number is the highest peak flow number you can achieve over a 2-week period when your asthma is under good control. Good control is when you feel good and do not have any asthma symptoms.

*continues*

continued

Each patient's asthma is different, and your best peak flow may be higher or lower than the peak flow of someone of your same height, weight, and sex. This means that it is important for you to find you own personal best peak flow number. Your medicine plan needs to be based on your own personal best peak flow number.

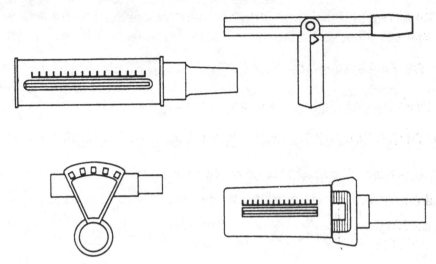

*There are a variety of peak flow meters.*

To find out your personal best peak flow number, take peak flow readings:

- every day for 2 weeks
- mornings and early afternoons or evenings (when you wake up and between 12:00 and 2:00 p.m.)
- before and after taking inhaled beta$_2$-agonist (*if* you take this medicine)
- as instructed by your doctor

## THE PEAK FLOW ZONE SYSTEM

Once you know your personal best peak flow number, your doctor will give you the numbers that tell you what to do. The peak flow numbers are put into zones that are set up like a traffic light. This will help you know what to do when your peak flow number changes. For example:

**Green Zone** (80 to 100 percent of your personal best number) signals ***good control***. No asthma symptoms are present. You may take your medicines as usual.

**Yellow Zone** (50 to 79 percent of your personal best number) signals ***caution***. You may be having an episode of asthma that requires an increase in your medicines. Or your overall asthma may not be under control, and the doctor may need to change your medicine plan.

*continues*

continued

**Red Zone** (below 50 percent of your personal best number) signals *danger!* You must take a short-acting, inhaled beta$_2$-agonist right away and call your doctor immediately if your peak flow number does not return to the Yellow or Green Zone and stay in that zone.

Record your personal best peak flow number and peak flow zones at the top of "My Asthma Symptoms and Peak Flow Diary."

### USE THE DIARY TO KEEP TRACK OF YOUR PEAK FLOW

Write down your peak flow number on the diary every day, or as instructed by your doctor.

### ACTIONS TO TAKE WHEN PEAK FLOW NUMBERS CHANGE

- **PEFR goes more than 20 percent below your personal best (PEFR is in the Yellow Zone)**

  **ACTION:** Take an inhaled short-acting bronchodilator as prescribed by your doctor.

- **PEFR changes 20 percent or more between the morning and early afternoon or evening** (measure your PEFR before taking medicine)

  or

- **PEFR increases 20 percent or more when measured before and after taking an inhaled short-acting bronchodilator.**

  **ACTION:** Talk to your doctor about adding more medicine to control your asthma better (for example, an anti-inflammatory medication).

**NOTES:**

Source: "Nurses: Partners in Asthma Care," National Asthma Education and Prevention Program, National Heart, Lung, and Blood Institute, NIH Publication No. 95-3308, 1995.

# El medidor de flujo espiratorio máximo—
# Un termómetro para el asma

El medidor de flujo espiratorio máximo (flujómetro) para un paciente con asma es como un termómetro para un paciente con fiebre. Los medidores de flujo espiratorio máximo ayudan a determinar en qué medida están abiertas sus vías respiratorias, en vez de adivinar con sólo cómo se siente.

En algunos casos cuando usted no se siente bien, se puede sentir con fiebre o "acalenturado" pero cuando toma su temperatura con un termómetro, es normal. Con el asma siente algunas veces que su respiración está "cerrada" o su tórax se puede sentir pesado pero usted tiene una función pulmonar normal. Su medidor de flujo espiratorio máximo le ayuda a determinar si su sensación de tórax cerrado es realmente un cambio de las vías respiratorias o no, del mismo modo en que el termómetro le ayuda a determinar si su sensación de calor es realmente fiebre.

Los pacientes se pueden beneficiar de varias maneras con el uso del medidor de flujo espiratorio máximo: para reconocer que el asma puede estar ocurriendo en la noche, para mejorar la percepción del asma, para identificar los factores que empeoran el asma, y para predecir el empeoramiento del asma.

### ¿Qué es un medidor de flujo espiratorio máximo?

Un medidor de flujo espiratorio máximo es un aparato sencillo, portátil y barato que mide el flujo de aire o la cifra de flujo espiratorio máximo (FEM). Hay varios medidores disponibles que varían muy poco en exactitud, durabilidad y precio. Si se usa adecuadamente, el medidor de flujo espiratorio máximo puede ser una herramienta valiosa en el manejo de su asma. Los medidores de flujo espiratorio máximo se pueden obtener sin receta, pero idealmente deben ser usados con la recomendación de un médico.

### USO DE UN MEDIDOR DE FLUJO ESPIRATORIO MÁXIMO

Los medidores de flujo espiratorio máximo pueden ser usados como herramientas para: (1) determinar la gravedad del asma; (2) verificar la respuesta al tratamiento durante un episodio agudo de asma; (3) observar-estudiar el progreso en el tratamiento de asma crónica y obtener información objetiva para cualquier posible ajuste en el tratamiento; (4) detectar el empeoramiento en la función pulmonar y de este modo evitar una probable exacerbación seria en el asma con intervención temprana; y (5) diagnosticar asma inducida por ejercicio.

Una de las funciones más importantes del medidor de flujo espiratorio máximo es el ayudar al paciente y al especialista en alergias a evaluar la gravedad del asma. La caída de las lecturas del flujo espiratorio máximo antes de los síntomas de asma es un aviso de que se tiene que hacer un ajuste. La señal temprana de alerta puede significar el agregar un medicamento o hacer otros

*continúa*

continuación

cambios en el plan de tratamiento. Cuanto más temprana sea la señal de alarma y más rápido se corrija el problema, se tomará menos tiempo y menos medicamentos para regresar los pulmones a la normalidad. Algunos pacientes con asma han establecido un programa de respaldo con su especialista en alergias, para saber qué medicamento agregar si su flujo máximo disminuye por debajo de cierto nivel. Aunque los medidores de flujo máximo no son un sustituto para las medidas espirométricas en la oficina del médico, son muy útiles para estos propósitos.

## SE NECESITA UN ENTRENAMIENTO ADECUADO

Con la observación casera del flujo espiratorio máximo, es esencial que el paciente siga algunas guías importantes: (1) aprender de un profesional hábil cómo usar adecuadamente un medidor de flujo espiratorio máximo; (2) aprender cómo y cuándo anotar (en una tabla) las lecturas del flujo espiratorio máximo; y (3) aprender qué hacer si descienden las lecturas del flujo espiratorio máximo.

Los padres de niños pequeños también deberán aprender estas guías. Los pacientes deben traer sus medidores de flujo espiratorio máximo al consultorio médico para verificar la exactitud del aparato así como para reverificar el uso adecuado del medidor.

## ASMA EN LA NOCHE

El asma usualmente empeora en la noche, aunque algunos pacientes duermen durante la noche sin estar alerta de niveles más bajos de flujo espiratorio máximo. Cuando dormimos, existe una disminución en la cantidad de oxígeno en la sangre, pero en asmáticos, esta caída de oxígeno puede suceder más frecuentemente y durar más tiempo. La gravedad del asma en la noche puede ser captada con un medidor de flujo pico. Usted no tiene que despertarse para usar el medidor. Compare la lectura de la mañana con la lectura de la noche anterior para determinar el grado de asma nocturna. Una disminución de 15% o mayor de la medida de la noche anterior puede indicar asma nocturna, lo cual puede comentarle a su especialista en alergias para corregirla.

## HERRAMIENTA OBJETIVA DE MEDIDA

El uso regular de monitores del flujo espiratorio máximo ha demostrado que ayuda a los pacientes a tener una idea más clara de cómo están funcionando sus pulmones. Sin medidas objetivas, es difícil determinar qué factores "desencadenantes" pueden causar que la función pulmonar empeore. Para señalar con exactitud los desencadenantes de asma, puede escribir las lecturas de flujo espiratorio máximo antes y después de la exposición a alergenos, irritantes ocupacionales, ejercicio, u otros eventos potencialmente asmagénicos. Las lecturas del flujo espiratorio máximo durante las diferentes estaciones del año pueden ayudar a identificar problemas que pueden estar causados por pólenes, aire frío o seco. Los múltiples beneficios del uso adecuado de los medidores del flujo espiratorio máximo hace que valga la pena considerarlos para cualquier paciente asmático, especialmente si el asma ha sido difícil de manejar.

*continúa*

continuación

## PASOS PARA USAR EL MEDIDOR DE FLUJO ESPIRATORIO MÁXIMO

Existen varios pasos para usar adecuadamente un medidor de flujo espiratorio máximo. Usted debe soplar fuertemente en el medidor para obtener la mejor lectura posible y repetir este intento tres veces. Anote la mejor de las tres medidas. Las tres medidas tienen que ser casi iguales para demostrar que se hizo un buen intento en cada una. Esto es especialmente importante cuando los padres están evaluando el asma del niño.

Así también, es útil el anotar lecturas antes y después del uso de broncodilatadores inhalados. Dos símbolos diferentes como "X" y "O", pueden ser usados para llevar un cuadro de estas lecturas cada mañana y noche. Un especialista en alergias puede obtener bastante información revisando estas lecturas. Esto también le ayudará a obtener mayor conciencia de su función pulmonar.

Teniendo una tabla de las lecturas del flujo espiratorio máximo, con cada día anotado en una columna, le ayuda a ver cómo se está comportando el asma. Gráficas para trazar las lecturas del flujo espiratorio máximo vienen frecuentemente con los aparatos y pueden ser fotocopiadas para su uso regular.

Tenga en mente que existen algunas guías generales que seguir cuando se esté usando el medidor de flujo espiratorio máximo:

1. No son necesarias las pinzas nasales;
2. Asegúrese que el aparato marque cero o se encuentre en su nivel base;
3. De pie (al menos que esté incapacitado, en este caso la posición será la misma para todas las maniobras);
4. Tome una inspiración profunda tan rápidamente como le sea posible;
5. Coloque el medidor en la boca y cierre los labios alrededor de la boquilla;
6. Sople tan fuertemente y rápidamente como le sea posible (uno a dos segundos);
7. No tosa ni deje que la lengua obstruya la boquilla;
8. Anote el valor obtenido;
9. Repita el procedimiento dos veces más;
10. Observe el mayor de los tres números obtenidos y anótelo en su diario.

Los medidores de flujo necesitan cuidado. Siga las instrucciones de limpieza que se encuentran dentro de las unidades. Esto ayuda a asegurar la exactitud.

## ESTABLEZCA SU "MEJOR MARCA" DE FLUJO ESPIRATORIO MÁXIMO

Aunque su valor predecible de flujo espiratorio máximo "normal", está determinado según su altura, edad y sexo, es preferible estimar el control del asma comparando los registros diarios de flujo espiratorio con la lectura de su "mejor marca". Esta se define como la medida más alta que usted puede alcanzar a la mitad de un buen día, después de usar su broncodilatador inhalado.

*continúa*

continuación

Su especialista en alergias puede ayudarle a determinar su mejor marca usando un régimen médico fuerte para normalizar la función pulmonar determinado por medidas de alta sensibilidad en su consultorio llamadas espirometría. Los valores pueden entonces correlacionarse con su propio medidor de flujo espiratorio máximo para establecer las metas de tratamiento de su asma. En general, los objetivos del flujo espiratorio máximo en niños no deben disminuir y, de hecho, deben reajustarse hacia arriba anualmente de acuerdo al crecimiento.

## MANEJO DEL ASMA: SISTEMA DEL SEMÁFORO

Una vez que se ha establecido la mejor marca de flujo espiratorio máximo, se debe esforzar por mantenerlo dentro del 80% de este número. Se ha establecido un sistema de semáforo como una guía general para ayudar a los pacientes en el manejo del asma.

**Zona verde:** FEM (PEFR) 80% A 100% de su mejor marca. "SIN PROBLEMA"- deberá estar relativamente asintomático y puede mantener su régimen médico actual. Si se encuentra con tratamiento médico crónico y su flujo espiratorio máximo se encuentra constantemente en la zona verde con una mínima variación, su médico debe considerar la disminución gradual de sus medicamentos diarios.

**Zona amarilla:** FEM 50-80% de su mejor marca. "PRECAUCIÓN"- el asma está empeorando. Es recomendable un aumento temporal de los medicamentos para el asma. Si se encuentra con medicamentos de uso crónico, probablemente necesite incrementarse el tratamiento de mantenimiento. Póngase en contacto con su médico para regular su tratamiento.

**Zona roja:** FEM DEBAJO DEL 50% de su mejor marca. "PELIGRO"- está fracasando el control del asma. Utilice su broncodilatador inhalado. Si el flujo espiratorio máximo regresa a la zona amarilla, llame a su médico inmediatamente, debe emplearse tratamiento agresivo bajo dirección médica. En cualquier caso, debe aumentarse el tratamiento de mantenimiento.

Estas zonas de semáforo son solamente una guía general diseñada para simplificar el manejo del asma. El éxito del control del asma depende de la relación entre el paciente y el médico. La comunicación abierta y el intercambio de información puede aumentarse con el monitoreo del flujo espiratorio máximo y los informes. Su médico puede usar estos datos objetivos para diseñar y ajustar de un modo óptimo su tratamiento de asma.

Courtesy of American Academy of Allergy, Asthma and Immunology, 1-800-822-2762, www.aaaai.org.

# Peak Flow Chart

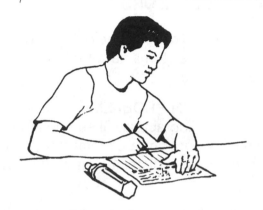

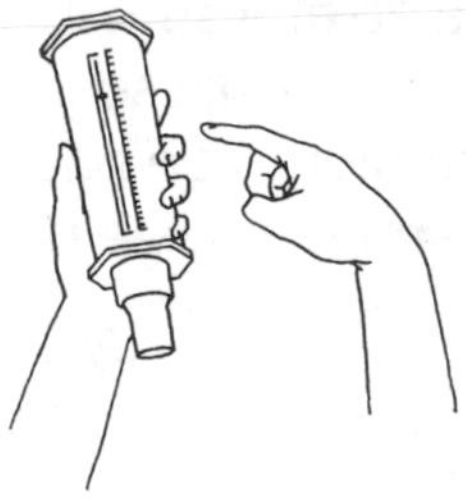

Name: _____

Doctor: _____

Date: _____

## How to use a peak flow chart at home.

1. Find your peak flow number in the morning and evening.
2. Each morning and each evening, blow three times.
3. After each blow, mark the spot where the marker stopped.
4. Put the meter next to the peak flow chart to help you find the spot to mark.
5. Circle the highest of the three numbers. That is your peak flow number.

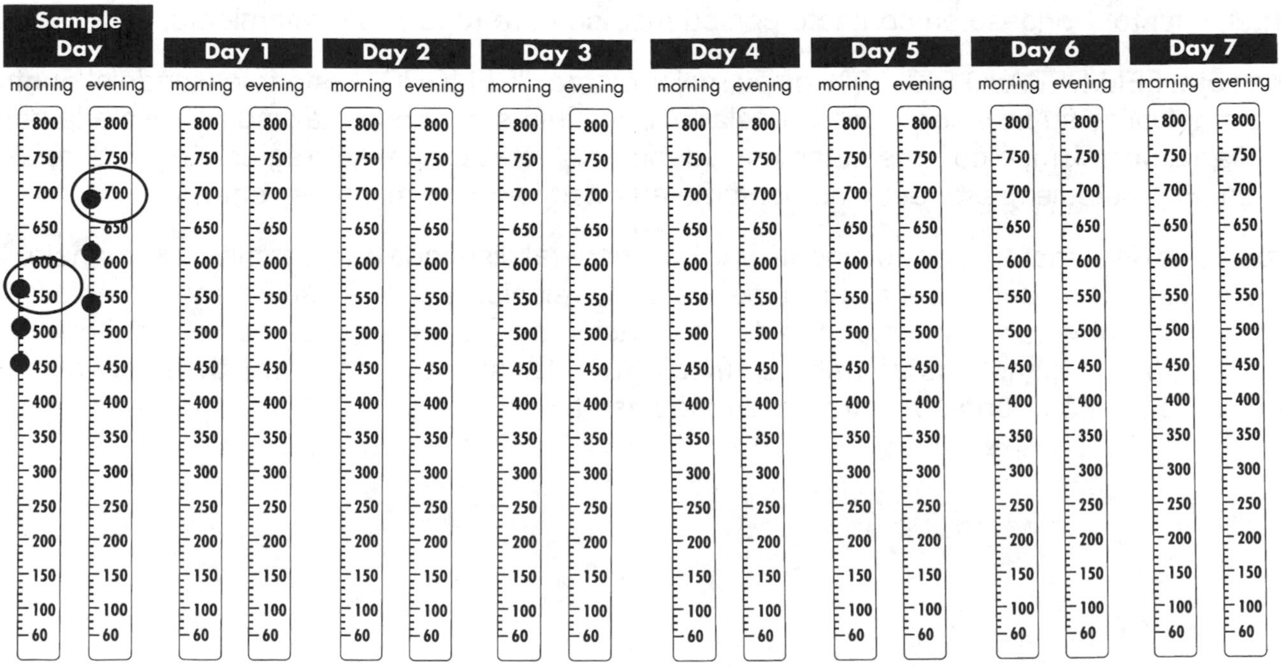

| Sample Day | | Day 1 | | Day 2 | | Day 3 | | Day 4 | | Day 5 | | Day 6 | | Day 7 | |
|---|---|---|---|---|---|---|---|---|---|---|---|---|---|---|---|
| morning | evening | morning | evening | morning | evening | morning | evening | morning | evening | morning | evening | morning | evening | morning | evening |

(Each column shows a vertical scale marked: 800, 750, 700, 650, 600, 550, 500, 450, 400, 350, 300, 250, 200, 150, 100, 60)

On the Sample Day morning column, marks at 450, 500, 550 (circled); evening column, marks at 550, 600, 700 (circled).

Source: "Global Initiative for Asthma, What You and Your Family Can Do about Asthma," National Heart, Lung, and Blood Institute, December 1995.

# My Asthma Symptoms and Peak Flow Diary

_____ **My predicted peak flow**          _____ **My personal best peak flow**

_____ **My Green (Good Control) Zone**    _____ **My Yellow (Caution) Zone**    _____ **My Red (Danger) Zone**
80–100% of personal best          50–79% of personal best          below 50% of personal best

| Date: | a.m. | p.m. | a.m. | p.m. | a.m. | p.m. | a.m. | p.m. | a.m. | p.m. | a.m. | p.m. | a.m. | p.m. |
|---|---|---|---|---|---|---|---|---|---|---|---|---|---|---|
| Peak Flow Reading | | | | | | | | | | | | | | |
| No Asthma Symptoms | | | | | | | | | | | | | | |
| Mild Asthma Symptoms | | | | | | | | | | | | | | |
| Moderate Asthma Symptoms | | | | | | | | | | | | | | |
| Serious Asthma Symptoms | | | | | | | | | | | | | | |
| Medicine Used To Stop Symptoms | | | | | | | | | | | | | | |
| Urgent Visit to the Doctor | | | | | | | | | | | | | | |

## DIRECTIONS

1. Take your peak flow reading every morning (a.m.) when you wake up and every afternoon or evening (p.m.). Try to take your peak flow readings at the same time each day. If you take an inhaled beta$_2$-agonist medicine, take your peak flow reading **before** taking that medicine. Write down the highest reading of three tries in the box that says **Peak Flow Reading**.
2. Look at the box at the top of this sheet to see whether your number is in the Green, Yellow, or Red Zone.

*continues*

continued

3. In the space below the date and time, put an "X" in the box that matches the symptoms you have when you record your peak flow reading. See description of symptom categories below.

4. Look at your Asthma Management Plan for what to do when your number is in one of the zones or when you have asthma symptoms.

5. Put an "X" in the box beside "medicine used to stop symptoms" if you took **extra** asthma medicine to stop your symptoms.

6. If you made any visit to your doctor's office, emergency department, or hospital for treatment of an asthma episode, put an "X" in the box marked "urgent visit to the doctor." Tell the doctor if you went to the emergency department or hospital.

| | | |
|---|---|---|
| **No symptoms** | = | No symptoms (no wheeze, cough, chest tightness, or shortness of breath) even with normal physical activity |
| **Mild symptoms** | = | Symptoms during physical activity, but not at rest. Symptoms do not keep you from sleeping or being active |
| **Moderate symptoms** | = | Symptoms while at rest; symptoms may keep you from sleeping or being active |
| **Severe symptoms** | = | Severe symptoms at rest (wheeze may be absent); symptoms cause problems walking or talking; muscles in neck or between ribs are pulled in when breathing |

Source: "Nurses: Partners in Asthma Care," National Asthma Education and Prevention Program, National Heart, Lung, and Blood Institute, NIH Publication No. 95-3308, 1995.

# How To Stop Asthma Attacks from Happening

**Many things can start asthma attacks**

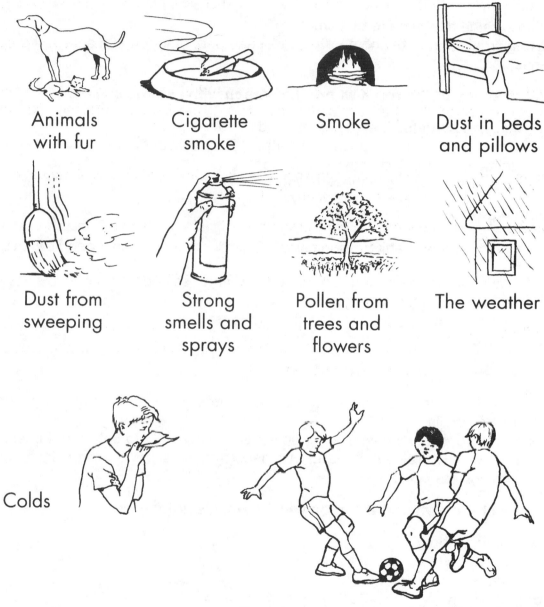

Animals with fur

Cigarette smoke

Smoke

Dust in beds and pillows

Dust from sweeping

Strong smells and sprays

Pollen from trees and flowers

The weather

Colds

Running, sports, and working hard

Sometimes these things are called asthma triggers.

*continues*

continued

## Keep things out of the home that start asthma attacks.

- Many people with asthma are allergic to animals with fur. Keep animals outside. Give away pets.
- No smoking inside. Get help to quit smoking.
- Keep strong smells out of the home. No soap, shampoo, or lotion that smells like perfume. No incense.

## Make special changes to the room where the person with asthma sleeps.

- Take out rugs and carpets. They get dusty and moldy.
- Take out soft chairs, cushions, and extra pillows. They collect dust.
- Do not let animals on the bed or in the bedroom.
- No smoking or strong smells in the bedroom.

## Keep the bed simple.

Dust collects in the mattress, blankets, and pillows. This dust bothers most people with asthma.

- Put special dust-proof covers with zippers on the mattress and pillow.
- Do not use a pillow or a mattress made of straw.
- A simple sleeping mat may be better than a mattress.
- Wash sheets and blankets often in very hot water. Put them in the sun to dry.

## Use windows to keep the air fresh and clean.

- Open windows wide when it is hot or stuffy, when there is smoke from cooking, and when there are strong smells.
- If you heat with wood or kerosene, keep a window open a little to get rid of fumes.
- Close windows when the air outside is full of exhaust from cars, pollution from factories, dust, or pollen from flowers and trees.

## Plan to do these chores when the person with asthma is not there:

- Sweep, vacuum, or dust
- Paint
- Spray for insects
- Use strong cleaners
- Cook strong smelling foods
- Air out the house before the person with asthma returns

If there is no one to help, people with asthma can use a mask or scarf when they sweep or dust.

Source: "Global Initiative for Asthma, What You and Your Family Can Do about Asthma," National Heart, Lung, and Blood Institute, December 1995.

# How To Stay Away from Things That Make Your Asthma Worse

Because you have asthma, your airways are very sensitive. They may react to things that can cause asthma attacks or episodes. Staying away from such things will help you keep your asthma from getting worse.

- Ask your doctor to help you find out what makes your asthma worse. Discuss the ways to stay away from these things. The tips listed below will help you.
- Ask the doctor for help in deciding which actions will help the most to reduce your asthma symptoms. Carry out these actions first. Discuss the results of your efforts with the doctor.

### TIPS FOR PEOPLE WITH ASTHMA

### House-Dust Mites

The following actions should help you control house-dust mites:

- Encase your mattress and box spring in an airtight cover.
- Either encase your pillow or wash it in hot water once a week every week.
- Wash your bed covers, clothes, and stuffed toys once a week in hot water (130°F).

The following actions will also help you control dust mites—but they are not essential:

- Reduce indoor humidity to less than 50 percent. Use a dehumidifier if needed.
- Remove carpets from your bedroom.
- Do not sleep or lie on upholstered furniture. Replace with vinyl, leather, or wood furniture.
- Remove carpets that are laid on concrete.
- Stay out of a room while it is being vacuumed.
- If you must vacuum, one or more of the following things can be done to reduce the amount of dust you breathe in: (1) Use a dust mask. (2) Use a central vacuum cleaner with the collecting bag outside the home. (3) Use double-wall vacuum cleaner bags and exhaust-port HEPA (high-efficiency particulate air) filters.

### Animals

Some children are allergic to the dried flakes of skin, saliva, or urine from warm-blooded pets. Warm-blooded pets include ALL dogs, cats, birds, and rodents. The length of a pet's hair does not matter. Here are some tips for those allergic to animals:

- Remove the animal from the home or school classroom.
- Choose a pet without fur or feathers (such as a fish or a snake).

*continues*

continued

- If you must have a warm-blooded pet, keep the pet out of your bedroom at all times. Keeping the pet outside of the home is even better.
- If there is forced-air heating in the home with a pet, close the air ducts in your bedroom.
- Wash the pet weekly in warm water.
- Do not visit homes that have pets. If you must visit such places, take asthma medicine (cromolyn is often preferred) before going.
- Do not buy or use products made with feathers. Use pillows and comforters stuffed with synthetic fibers like polyester. Also, do not use pillows, bedding, and furniture stuffed with kapok (silky fibers from the seed pods of the silk-cotton tree).
- Use a vacuum cleaner fitted with a HEPA filter.
- Wash hands and change clothes as soon as you can after being in contact with pets.

### Cockroaches

Some people are allergic to the droppings of roaches.

- Use insect sprays, but have someone else spray when you are outside of the home. Air out the home for a few hours after spraying. Roach traps may also help.
- All homes in multiple-family dwellings (apartments, condominiums, and housing projects) must be treated to get rid of roaches.

### Tobacco Smoke

- Do not smoke.
- Do not allow smoking in the home. Have household members smoke outside.
- Encourage family members to quit smoking. Ask your doctor or nurse for help on how to quit.
- Choose no-smoking areas in restaurants, hotels, and other public buildings.

### Wood Smoke

- Do not use a wood-burning stove to heat the home.
- Do not use kerosene heaters.

### Strong Odors and Sprays

- Do not stay in your home when it is being painted. Use latex rather than oil-based paint.
- Try to stay away from perfume, talcum powder, hair spray, and products like these.
- Use household cleaning products that do not have strong smells or scents.
- Reduce strong cooking odors (especially frying) by using an exhaust fan and opening windows.

*continues*

continued

## Colds and Infections

- Talk to your doctor about flu shots.
- Stay away from people with colds or the flu.
- Do not take over-the-counter cold remedies, such as antihistamines and cough syrup, unless you speak to your doctor first.

## Exercise

- Make a plan with your doctor that allows you to exercise without symptoms. For example, take inhaled beta$_2$-agonist or cromolyn less than 30 minutes before exercising.
- Do not exercise during the afternoon when air pollution levels are highest.
- Warm up before doing exercise and cool down afterward.

## Weather

- Wear a scarf over your mouth and nose in cold weather. Or pull a turtleneck or scarf over your nose on windy or cold days.
- Dress warmly in the winter or on windy days.

## Pollens

During times of high pollen counts

- Stay indoors during the midday and afternoon when pollen counts are highest.
- Keep windows closed in cars and homes. Use air conditioning if you can.
- Pets should either stay outdoors or indoors. Pets should not be allowed to go in and out of the home. This prevents your pet from bringing pollen inside.
- Do not mow the grass. But if you must mow, wear a pollen filter mask.

## Mold (Outdoor)

- Avoid sources of molds (wet leaves, garden debris, stacked wood).
- Avoid standing water or areas of poor drainage.

**REMEMBER: Making these changes will help keep asthma episodes from starting. These actions can also reduce your need for asthma medicines.**

Source: "Nurses: Partners in Asthma Care," National Asthma Education and Prevention Program, National Heart, Lung, and Blood Institute, NIH Publication No. 95-3308, 1995.

# Removing House Dust and Other Allergic Irritants from Your Home

House dust is not dust that blows in from out-of-doors. Instead, house dust is produced indoors from fibers and the breakdown of plant and animal material used in the home. These plant and animal materials include feathers, cotton, wool, jute, hemp, animal hairs, etc. They can be found in such items as stuffing in mattresses, pillows, quilts, upholstered furniture, and carpets.

The components of house dust also may include human skin scales, animal dander and saliva, and a large variety of molds. Other allergy triggers found in the house are proteins from cockroaches and microscopic dust mites. These mites, which are related to spiders, produce allergenic proteins, which are one of the major triggers of asthma and other allergic reactions.

House-dust mite allergy is especially troublesome in homes where the indoor humidity is high or in houses at a low altitude. Dust mites can be found throughout the house, but they especially thrive where human dander is located, such as on mattresses, pillows, bed covers, upholstered furniture, and carpeting.

Symptoms of house dust allergy may include a blocked or runny nose with sneezing (particularly in the morning), watery eyes, occasional itching, rashes, coughing, and wheezing. Sometimes these symptoms may appear together but often individuals have one symptom only (e.g., asthma) and may not realize they are allergic to house dust.

## HOW TO REDUCE DUST IN THE HOME

Indoor environmental control is very important and effective in reducing allergic triggers. The bedroom is an important room to begin with, because more time is spent in the bedroom than any other room in the house. Here are some ways to reduce dust and other irritants in your home environment:

### Bedrooms

Smooth, uncluttered, easily cleaned surfaces are recommended. Small objects, such as knick-knacks, books, records, tapes, stereos, televisions, and stuffed animals should be placed in drawers or closed cabinets. Avoid using your bedroom as a library or study room.

### Mattresses

Encase mattresses in airtight covers. Controlling dust mites in mattresses requires either regular vacuuming or putting them in dust-free casings. The easier solution is to place zippered, air-tight plastic or special allergen-proof fabric casings on pillows, mattresses, and box springs. Water-

*continues*

continued

beds do not have this problem, but the mattress pad on top of the waterbed should be washed regularly.

## Bedding

Bedding must be washable and should be washed weekly in hot water. This is necessary since washing with cool water does not kill dust mites. Comforters and pillows made of down feathers, kapok, and cotton should be replaced with items made from synthetic fibers such as dacron or orlon. Comforters and pillows should be washed regularly, and synthetic pillows should be replaced every two to three years.

## Carpeting

Where possible, carpeting should be removed, since house-dust mites, mold spores, animal dander, and other allergens are abundant in carpeting. Hardwood or linoleum is much better for those with allergies. Carpeting laid over concrete floors contains especially high levels of dust mites because of the increased humidity.

## Vacuuming

Cleaning is essential, but vacuuming with a standard or water-filtered vacuum cleaner stirs dust up into the air. Allergic individuals should wear a dust mask while vacuuming or use a vacuum with a HEPA filter. Upholstered furniture should be vacuumed, and other surfaces should be mopped or wiped. Regular weekly house cleaning is suggested.

## Humidity/Air Conditioning

Controlling the indoor relative humidity to below 50% is important to reduce the growth of dust mites and mold. Central air conditioning is the most effective way of controlling humidity. Window units may be effective, but it is important to clean the filters on a regular basis. Air conditioning cleans and cools the indoor air and keeps the outside air outdoors.

This helps to reduce exposure to outdoor pollens and molds. Avoid window fans because they can help bring high levels of pollens and molds into the house. Swamp coolers should also be avoided, as they increase humidity to the range favorable to mites and molds.

## Chemical Agents

Chemical agents may kill the dust mites and/or reduce dust mite antigens in the house.

*continues*

continued

## Indoor Molds

Indoor molds thrive in areas of the house with increased humidity (moisture). Dehumidifiers are helpful in damp basements, but generally do not control humidity throughout the house. Basements, bathrooms, and kitchens need ventilation and consistent cleaning to help keep mold growth to a minimum. Mold killers, including chlorine bleach, TSP, and household cleaners help keep surfaces clear of mold. Other sources of mold are cold water humifiers, carpeting, plants, garbage containers, rotting flooring, window sills, damp firewood, and water-damaged wallpaper.

## Air-Cleaning Devices

The most effective way to reduce indoor allergens is to remove or control the source of allergens. Filtering the air to remove airborne allergens is an additional step that can help. Several filtering devices are available, and some can be used in conjunction with an existing forced air cooling and heating system. Mechanical filters using standard disposable fiberglass filters should be changed monthly. Permanent filters with baffles should be cleaned periodically. The most effective filter is a high-efficiency particulate (HEPA) filter that also mechanically cleans air.

Another device that can be used is an electric filter using an electrostatic precipitator. These filters require frequent cleaning of the plates and may produce irritating ozone if they are not well maintained.

Freestanding air cleaners using HEPA or electrostatic precipitators are available, although it is not certain how much they help. Two factors should be considered before purchasing one of these units: whether it can clean and circulate significant amounts of clean air, and whether allergens that the individual is sensitive to are prevalent in indoor air.

## Animal Dander

Individuals with animal allergies react to proteins from the animal's dander, urine, and/or saliva, which spread throughout the house. Removal of the animal is the most effective control measure, but this may not give immediate, total relief since animal allergens can be present in the house for months after removal. With cats, the main problem is with the protein in their saliva. Studies have shown that bathing the cat weekly may reduce the amount of dander and dried saliva deposited on carpeting, bedding, and elsewhere. Allergens from small animals such as mice and gerbils are found in their urine, so the cage litter is the source of the problem.

## Odors and Fumes

It is important that allergic patients avoid other irritants that can be found in the house, including tobacco smoke, aerosols, and cleaning products with strong odors.

*continues*

continued

## CONCLUSION

Indoor environmental control measures should focus on the sites where allergens are produced and accumulate. Allergic patients should know which specific allergens provoke their symptoms. Your allergist can help you to determine this. This is important, because environmental control measures for animals, dust mites, molds, and cockroaches differ.

Making these indoor environmental changes may take time. An allergy sufferer should write down a priority list and make changes over a period of months. These progressive changes will produce an indoor environment that is less allergenic, easier to clean, and healthier for the whole family.

## NOTES:

Courtesy of American Academy of Allergy Asthma and Immunology, 1-800-822-2762, www.aaaai.org.

# Desencadenantes de asma

## ALERGENOS

Los alergenos son desencadenantes importantes de asma. Estos son algunos ejemplos de alergenos intra y extramuros.

- Polen
- Hongos
- Caspas de animales
- Polvo casero/ácaros del polvo
- Cucarachas
- Algunos alimentos

## INFECCIONES VIRALES

Las infecciones virales de las vías respiratorias actúan frecuentemente como un desencadenante importante. Esto se verifica especialmente en niños pequeños con asma. Las infecciones virales producen una irritación agregada en las vías respiratorias, nariz, garganta, pulmones y senos paranasales. Esta irritación precede frecuentemente a los ataques de asma. No se sabe el mecanismo biológico exacto de este proceso.

## SINUSITIS

La sinusitis, que es una inflamación de los senos paranasales, frecuentementese inicia como una infección de vías aéreas superiores. Los síntomas en la niñez incluyen sibilancias, descarga retronasal, tos nocturna y ganglios inflamados. Los adolescentes y adultos pueden presentar dolor de cabeza, sensación de presión en los senos paranasales o dolor. El asma puede agravarse por el paso de moco a través de la nariz, garganta y bronquios.

## IRRITANTES

Los irritantes pueden ser desencadenantes importantes de asma. Algunos ejemplos son:

1. Olores fuertes y aerosoles tales como perfumes, limpiadores para la casa, humos de la cocina (especialmente frituras), pinturas y barnices;
2. Otros químicos como carbón, polvo de gis o talco;
3. Contaminantes ambientales;
4. Humo de tabaco;
5. Cambios de clima (incluyendo cambios de temperatura, presión barométrica, humedad y vientos fuertes) todos probablemente afectan e irritan las vías respiratorias.

*continúa*

continuación

## HUMO DE TABACO Y MADERA

El humo de tabaco, ya sea por inhalación directa o pasiva, tiene efectos dañinos en las vías respiratorias y es especialmente irritante para pacientes asmáticos. Se ha reportado un aumento en la incidencia de asma en niños de madres que fuman. Nadie debería fumar en casa de un paciente asmático.

El humo de calentadores que queman madera y de chimeneas puede ser extremadamente irritante para asmáticos a causa de la liberación de químicos tales como el dióxido de sulfuro. Se debe mantener buena ventilación si se usan calentadores y chimeneas, pero si es posible es mejor evitarlos.

## EJERCICIO

El ejercicio también puede desencadenar un ataque asmático. Se estima que el 85% de asmáticos alérgicos tienen síntomas de sibilancias después del ejercicio. La inhalación de aire frío y seco parece ser un fuerte desencadenante de asma. La carrera de larga distancia, una actividad extenuante y prolongada, es la más probable de inducir asma y la natación es la menos probable.

## REFLUJO GASTROESOFAGICO

El reflujo gastroesofágico es una condición caracterizada por reflujo persistente de ácidos estomacales, común en personas con asma. Los síntomas pueden incluir agruras, eruptos, y regurgitaciones (especialmente en lactantes). El asma nocturna es común.

## EXPOSICION INDUSTRIAL U OCUPACIONAL A IRRITANTES QUIMICOS DURANTE EL TRABAJO

En los Estados Unidos varios estudios indican que el asma puede ser empeorada o causada por exposición ocupacional a vapores, polvo, gases o humos.

Típicamente el asma ocupacional mejora cuando la persona se encuentra lejos de su trabajo por varios días ej., fines de semana y vacaciones.

## SENSIBILIDAD A MEDICAMENTOS

Del 5 al 20% de pacientes asmáticos adultos pueden presentar un ataque de asma como resultado de sensibilidad o alergias a medicamentos. Los medicamentos que se sabe pueden inducir un ataque de asma incluyen:

1. Aspirina;
2. Otros antiinflamatorios no esteroideos en pacientes con sensibilidad a la aspirina como ibuprofeno, indometacina, naproxeno, etc.;

*continúa*

continuación

3. Sulfitos usados como conservadores de alimentos y bebidas;
4. Beta bloqueadores (medicamentos frecuentemente usados para tratamientos de enfermedades cardiacas hipertensión y migraña).

Los asmáticos deben consultar a su médico, antes de tomar cualquier medicamento, incluyendo medicamentos que se venden sin receta en la farmacia.

## ANSIEDAD EMOCIONAL

La ansiedad y el stress nervioso causan fatiga y pueden aumentar los síntomas de asma y agravar un ataque. Estos factores psicológicos por sí solos no provocan asma y se consideran más como un efecto que como una causa.

# Patient Self-Assessment Form for Environmental and Other Factors That Can Make Asthma Worse

Patient Name: _____    Date: _____

Do you cough, wheeze, have chest tightness, or feel short of breath year-round? (If no, go to next question) ............................    No ____ Yes ____
If yes:
- Are there pets or animals in your home, school, or day care? ........    No ____ Yes ____
- Is there moisture or dampness in any room of your home? .........    No ____ Yes ____
- Have you seen mold or smelled musty odors any place in your home?    No ____ Yes ____
- Have you seen cockroaches in your home? ......................    No ____ Yes ____
- Do you use a humidifier or swamp cooler in your home? ...........    No ____ Yes ____

Does your coughing, wheezing, chest tightness, or shortness of breath get worse at certain times of the year? (If no, go to next question) .....    No ____ Yes ____
If yes:
Do your symptoms get worse in the:
- Early spring? (Trees) ....................................    No ____ Yes ____
- Late spring? (Grasses) ...................................    No ____ Yes ____
- Late summer to autumn? (Weeds) ...........................    No ____ Yes ____
- Summer and fall? (*Alternaria, Cladosporium*) ...................    No ____ Yes ____

Do you smoke? .............................................    No ____ Yes ____
Does anyone smoke at home, work, or day care? ..................    No ____ Yes ____

Is a wood-burning stove or fireplace used in your home? ...........    No ____ Yes ____
Are kerosene, oil, or gas stoves or heaters used without vents in your home? ................................................    No ____ Yes ____
Are you exposed to fumes or odors from cleaning agents, sprays, or other chemicals? .........................................    No ____ Yes ____

Do you cough or wheeze during the week, but not on weekends when away from work or school? .............................    No ____ Yes ____
Do your eyes and nose get irritated soon after you get to work or school? ................................................    No ____ Yes ____
Do your coworkers or classmates have symptoms like yours? ........    No ____ Yes ____
Are isocyanates, plant or animal products, smoke, gases, or fumes used where you work? ..........................................    No ____ Yes ____
Is it cold, hot, dusty, or humid where you work? ..................    No ____ Yes ____

*continues*

continued

Do you have a stuffy nose or postnasal drip, either at certain times of
  the year or year-round? . . . . . . . . . . . . . . . . . . . . . . . . . . . . . . . . . . .    No ____ Yes ____
Do you sneeze often or have itchy, watery eyes? . . . . . . . . . . . . . . . . . .    No ____ Yes ____

Do you have heartburn? . . . . . . . . . . . . . . . . . . . . . . . . . . . . . . . . . . . .    No ____ Yes ____
Does food sometimes come up into your throat? . . . . . . . . . . . . . . . . . .    No ____ Yes ____
Have you had coughing, wheezing, or shortness of breath at night in
  the past 4 weeks? . . . . . . . . . . . . . . . . . . . . . . . . . . . . . . . . . . . . .    No ____ Yes ____
Does your infant vomit, then cough or have wheezy cough at night?  . . .    No ____ Yes ____
Are these symptoms worse after feeding? . . . . . . . . . . . . . . . . . . . . . . .    No ____ Yes ____

Have you had wheezing, coughing, or shortness of breath after eating
  shrimp, dried fruit, or canned or processed potatoes? . . . . . . . . . . . .    No ____ Yes ____
After drinking beer or wine? . . . . . . . . . . . . . . . . . . . . . . . . . . . . . . . . .    No ____ Yes ____

Are you taking any prescription medicines or over-the-counter
  medicines? . . . . . . . . . . . . . . . . . . . . . . . . . . . . . . . . . . . . . . . . . . .    No ____ Yes ____
If yes, which ones? _____

Do you use eye drops? . . . . . . . . . . . . . . . . . . . . . . . . . . . . . . . . . . . .    No ____ Yes ____
Do you use any medicines that contain beta-blockers (e.g., blood
  pressure medicine)? . . . . . . . . . . . . . . . . . . . . . . . . . . . . . . . . . . . . .    No ____ Yes ____
Do you ever take aspirin or other nonsteroidal anti-inflammatory drugs
  (like ibuprofen)? . . . . . . . . . . . . . . . . . . . . . . . . . . . . . . . . . . . . . . . .    No ____ Yes ____
Have you ever had coughing, wheezing, chest tightness, or shortness
  of breath after taking any medication? . . . . . . . . . . . . . . . . . . . . . . . .    No ____ Yes ____

Do you cough, wheeze, have chest tightness, or feel shortness of breath
  during or after exercising? . . . . . . . . . . . . . . . . . . . . . . . . . . . . . . . .    No ____ Yes ____

Source: "Practical Guide for the Diagnosis and Management of Asthma" (Based on the *Expert Panel Report II: Guidelines for the Diagnosis and Management of Asthma*), NIH Publication No. 97-4053, National Heart, Lung, and Blood Institute, National Institutes of Health, October 1997.

# Talking to People about Asthma

It is important to talk about asthma to others. Family, friends, and teachers or coworkers can give you a lot of support if they know the facts and how they can help.

## WHEN YOU TALK ABOUT ASTHMA

- Do not make a big deal out of it, and do not encourage people to feel sorry for you.

- Explain that a person whose asthma is under control can perform just like other people.

- Explain that you know how to take care of asthma when you are having symptoms.

- Describe the steps you take to prevent and control symptoms. Tell them what, if anything, you would like them to do to help.

- Choose the right time to tell each person about asthma. For instance,
  —Tell teachers and coaches at the beginning of the school year.
  —Tell friends and coworkers in private, and when you are not having symptoms.

**NOTES:**

Source: "Teach Your Patients about Asthma," National Heart, Lung, and Blood Institute, October 1992.

# Check Your Asthma IQ

The following true-or-false statements test what you know about asthma. Be sure to read the correct answers and explanations on the back of this sheet.

T    F    1. Asthma is a common disease among children and adults in the United States.

T    F    2. Asthma is an emotional or psychological illness.

T    F    3. The way that parents raise their children can cause asthma.

T    F    4. Asthma episodes may cause breathing problems, but these episodes are not really harmful or dangerous.

T    F    5. Asthma episodes usually occur suddenly without warning.

T    F    6. Many different things can bring on an asthma episode.

T    F    7. Asthma cannot be cured, but it can be controlled.

T    F    8. There are different types of medicine to control asthma.

T    F    9. People with asthma have no way to monitor how well their lungs are functioning.

T    F   10. Both children and adults can have asthma.

T    F   11. Tobacco smoke can make an asthma episode worse.

T    F   12. People with asthma should not exercise.

Your Score: How many answers did you get correct?

| 11–12 correct | = Congratulations! You know a lot about asthma. Share this information with your family and friends. |
| 10–11 correct | = Very good. |
| Fewer than 10 correct | = Go over the answers and try to learn more about asthma. |

**Answers to the Asthma IQ Quiz**

1. **True.** Asthma is a common disease among children and adults in the United States, and it is increasing. About 10 million people have asthma, of whom 3 million are under 18 years of age.

*continues*

continued

2. **False.** Asthma is not an emotional or psychological disease, although strong emotions can sometimes make asthma worse. People with asthma have sensitive lungs that react to certain things, causing the airways to tighten, swell, and fill with mucus. The person then has trouble breathing and may cough and wheeze.

3. **False.** The way parents raise their children does not cause asthma. It is not caused by a poor parent-child relationship or by being overprotective.

4. **False.** Asthma episodes can be harmful. People can get very sick and need hospitalization. Some people have died from asthma episodes. Frequent asthma episodes, even if they are mild, may cause people to stop being active and living normal lives.

5. **False.** Sometimes an asthma episode may come on quite quickly. However, before a person has any wheezing or shortness of breath there are usually symptoms such as a cough, a scratchy throat, or tightness in the chest. Most patients learn to recognize these early symptoms and can take medicine to prevent a serious episode.

6. **True.** For most people with asthma, an episode can start from many different "triggers." Some of these things are pollen from trees or grasses; molds or house dust; weather changes; strong odors; cigarette smoke; and certain foods. Other triggers include being upset; laughing or crying hard; having a cold or the flu; or being near furry or feathered animals. Each person with asthma has an individual set of asthma "triggers."

7. **True.** There is no cure yet for asthma. However, asthma patients can control it to a large degree by:

   - Getting advice from a doctor who treats asthma patients
   - Learning to notice early signs of an asthma episode and to start treatment
   - Avoiding things that can cause asthma episodes
   - Taking medicine just as the doctor says
   - Knowing when to get medical help with a severe episode.

8. **True.** Several types of medicines are available to control asthma. Some people with mild asthma need to take medication only when they have symptoms. But most people need to take medicine every day to prevent symptoms and also to take medicine when symptoms do occur. A doctor needs to decide the best type of medicine for each patient and how often it should be taken. Asthma patients and their doctors need to work together to manage the disease.

9. **False.** People with asthma can monitor how well their lungs are functioning with a peak flow meter. This small device can be used at home, work, or school. The peak flow meter may show that the asthma is getting worse before the usual symptoms appear.

10. **True.** Both children and adults can have asthma. Sometimes, but not always, symptoms will go away as children get older. However, many children continue to have asthma

*continues*

continued

symptoms throughout adulthood. In some cases, symptoms of asthma are not recognized until a person is an adult.

11. **True.** Smoke from cigarettes, cigars, and pipes can bring on an asthma attack. Indoor smoky air from fireplaces and outdoor smog can make asthma worse. Some can also "set off" other triggers. Smokers should be asked not to smoke near someone with asthma. Moving to another room may help, but smoke travels room to room. No smoking is best for everyone!

12. **False.** Exercise is good for most people—with or without asthma. When asthma is under good control, people with asthma are able to play most sports. For people whose asthma is brought on by exercise, medicines can be taken before exercising to help avoid an episode. A number of Olympic medalists have asthma.

Source: "Check Your Asthma I.Q.," NIH Publication No. 92-1128, National Asthma Education and Prevention Program, National Heart, Lung, and Blood Institute, National Institutes of Health, October 1992.

# Worksheet: What To Expect From Your Asthma Treatment—The Goals

Put a checkmark next to each goal that you are meeting. Tell your doctor which goals you are meeting and which you are not. Do this at every visit.

- ☐ No symptoms or minor symptoms of asthma (symptoms include wheezing, coughing, shortness of breath, and chest tightness)

- ☐ Sleeping through the night without asthma symptoms

- ☐ No time off from school or work from asthma

- ☐ Full participation in physical activities

- ☐ No emergency room visits or stays in the hospital

- ☐ Little or no side effects from asthma medicine

**Do not accept having symptoms as normal.**

**Tell your doctor which goals you are meeting and which you are not. Do this at every visit.**
All of these goals can be met with long-term treatment. You need to work with your doctor to achieve every goal. If you are not meeting a goal, your treatment may simply need to be changed. Your doctor may ask for help from a specialist to achieve your goals. Ask about this.

Source: "What To Expect from Your Asthma Treatment: The Goals," NIH Publication No. 91-2664, U.S. Department of Health and Human Services, National Institutes of Health, September 1991.

# Patient Self-Assessment Form for Follow-Up Visits

Patient Name: _____     Date: _____

Please answer the questions below in the space provided on the right.

**Since your last visit:**

1. Has your asthma been any worse? . . . . . . . . . . . . . . . . . . . . . . . . .     No ____  Yes ____

2. Have there been any changes in your home, work, or school environment (such as a new pet, someone smoking)? . . . . . . . . . . . .     No ____  Yes ____

3. Have you had any times when your symptoms were a lot worse than usual? . . . . . . . . . . . . . . . . . . . . . . . . . . . . . . . . . . . . . . .     No ____  Yes ____

4. Has your asthma caused you to miss work or school or reduce or change your activities? . . . . . . . . . . . . . . . . . . . . . . . . . . . . . . .     No ____  Yes ____

5. Have you missed any regular doses of your medicines for any reason? . . . . . . . . . . . . . . . . . . . . . . . . . . . . . . . . . . . . . . . . . .     No ____  Yes ____

6. Have your medications caused you any problems? (shakiness, nervousness, bad taste, sore throat, cough, upset stomach)? . . . . .     No ____  Yes ____

7. Have you had any emergency room visits or hospital stays for asthma? . . . . . . . . . . . . . . . . . . . . . . . . . . . . . . . . . . . . . . . . . .     No ____  Yes ____

8. Has the cost of your asthma treatment kept you from getting the medicine or care you need for your asthma? . . . . . . . . . . . . . . . . . .     No ____  Yes ____

**In the past 2 weeks:**

9. Have you had a cough, wheezing, shortness of breath, or chest tightness during:

    - the day . . . . . . . . . . . . . . . . . . . . . . . . . . . . . . . . . . . . . . . . . .     No ____  Yes ____
    - night . . . . . . . . . . . . . . . . . . . . . . . . . . . . . . . . . . . . . . . . . . . . .     No ____  Yes ____
    - exercise or play? . . . . . . . . . . . . . . . . . . . . . . . . . . . . . . . . . . .     No ____  Yes ____

10. (If you use a peak flow meter) Did your peak flow go below 80 percent of your personal best? . . . . . . . . . . . . . . . . . . . . . . . . .     No ____  Yes ____

11. How many days have you used your inhaled quick-relief medicine? . . . . . . . . . . . . . . . . . . . . . . . . . . . . . . . . . . . . . . . . . .     Number of days _____

12. Have you been satisfied with the way your asthma has been? . . . . .     No ____  Yes ____

*continues*

continued

13. What are some concerns or questions you would like us to address at this visit?

_____

_____

_____

_____

For staff use.
☐ Peak Flow Technique
☐ MDI Technique
☐ Reviewed Action Plan:    ☐ Daily meds    ☐ Emergency meds

**NOTES:**

Source: "Practical Guide for the Diagnosis and Management of Asthma" (Based on the *Expert Panel Report II: Guidelines for the Diagnosis and Management of Asthma*), NIH Publication No. 97-4053, National Heart, Lung, and Blood Institute, National Institutes of Health, October 1997.

# Medicines for Asthma

**Most people with asthma need two kinds of asthma medicine**

1. Everyone with asthma needs a quick-relief medicine to stop asthma attacks.
2. Many people also need a preventive medicine every day to protect the lungs and keep asthma attacks from starting.

**Ask the doctor to write down what asthma medicines to take and when to take them**

- The doctor may use a medicine plan like the one below.

- Use the medicine plan to know what quick-relief medicines to take when you have an asthma attack.

- Use the medicine plan to help remember what preventive medicines to take every day.

- Use the medicine plan to see if you should take asthma medicine just before sports or working hard.

**ASTHMA MEDICINE PLAN**

Name: _____

Doctor: _____ Date: _____

Phone for doctor or clinic: _____

Phone for taxi or friend: _____

You can use the colors of a traffic light to help learn about your asthma medicines.
1. **Green** means **Go.** Use preventive medicine.
2. **Yellow** means **Caution.** Use quick-relief medicine.
3. **Red** means **Stop.** Get help from a doctor.

**1. Green—Go**

- breathing is good
- no cough or wheeze
- can work and play

Peak Flow Number
_____ to _____

Use preventive medicine.

| Medicine | How much to take | When to take it |
| --- | --- | --- |
| | | |
| | | |
| | | |

20 minutes before sports, use this medicine:

_____

*continues*

continued

- cough
- tight chest
- wheeze
- wake up at night

Peak Flow Number
_____ to _____

Cough        Wheeze

Tight        Wake up
chest        at night

- medicine is not helping
- breathing is hard and fast
- nose opens wide
- can't walk
- ribs show
- can't talk well

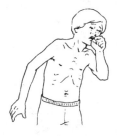

Peak Flow Number
_____ to _____

## 2. Yellow—Caution

Take quick-relief medicine to keep an asthma episode from getting bad.

| Medicine | How much to take | When to take it |
|----------|------------------|-----------------|
|          |                  |                 |
|          |                  |                 |
|          |                  |                 |
|          |                  |                 |
|          |                  |                 |
|          |                  |                 |

## 3. Red—Stop—Danger

**Get help from a doctor now!**

Take these medicines until you talk with the doctor.

| Medicine | How much to take | When to take it |
|----------|------------------|-----------------|
|          |                  |                 |
|          |                  |                 |
|          |                  |                 |
|          |                  |                 |

*continues*

continued

## Preventive medicines for asthma are safe to use every day

- You cannot become addicted to preventive medicines for asthma even if you use them for many years.
- Preventive medicine makes the swelling of the airways in the lungs go away.
- The doctor may tell you to take preventive medicine every day:
  —if you cough, wheeze, or have a tight chest more than once a week
  —if you wake up at night because of asthma
  —if you have many asthma episodes
  —if you have to use quick-relief medicine every day to stop asthma attacks

## Tell the doctor about any problems with your asthma medicines

- The doctor can change the asthma medicine or change how much you take. There are many asthma medicines.
- Go to the doctor 2 or 3 times a year for checkups so the doctor can see how well the asthma medicine works.
- Asthma may get better or it may get worse over the years. The doctor may need to change your asthma medicines.

## Asthma medicine can be taken in different ways

When asthma medicine is breathed in, it goes right to the airways in the lungs where it is needed. Inhalers for asthma come in many shapes. Most are sprays. Some use powder.

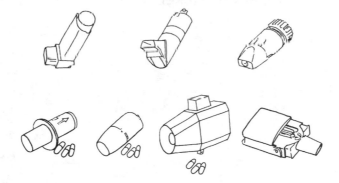

Asthma medicine also comes as pills and syrups.

## Be prepared—Always have asthma medicine.

- Set aside money for asthma medicine. Buy more before you run out.
- Always carry your quick-relief asthma medicine with you when you leave home.

Source: "Global Initiative for Asthma, What You and Your Family Can Do about Asthma," National Heart, Lung, and Blood Institute, December 1995.

# Asthma Medicines for _____

(Name of Patient)

**Date:** _____

| Medicine | Dose | Times to be taken | | When to take |
|---|---|---|---|---|
| | | | _____ | Every day |
| | | | _____ | When peak flow drops 10 to 20 percent |
| | | | _____ | For symptoms or signs of asthma |
| | | | _____ | Before exercise |
| | | | _____ | Before contact with triggers |
| | | | _____ | Other |

**Purpose:**

**Special instructions** (side effects, forgot medicine, etc.):

| Medicine | Dose | Times to be taken | | When to take |
|---|---|---|---|---|
| | | | _____ | Every day |
| | | | _____ | When peak flow drops 10 to 20 percent |
| | | | _____ | For symptoms or signs of asthma |
| | | | _____ | Before exercise |
| | | | _____ | Before contact with triggers |
| | | | _____ | Other |

**Purpose:**

**Special instructions** (side effects, forgot medicine, etc.):

*continues*

continued

| Medicine | Dose | Times to be taken | When to take |
|----------|------|-------------------|--------------|

**When to take**

_____ Every day

_____ When peak flow drops 10 to 20 percent

_____ For symptoms or signs of asthma

_____ Before exercise

_____ Before contact with triggers

_____ Other

**Purpose:**

**Special instructions** (side effects, forgot medicine, etc.):

---

| Medicine | Dose | Times to be taken | When to take |
|----------|------|-------------------|--------------|

**When to take**

_____ Every day

_____ When peak flow drops 10 to 20 percent

_____ For symptoms or signs of asthma

_____ Before exercise

_____ Before contact with triggers

_____ Other

**Purpose:**

**Special instructions** (side effects, forgot medicine, etc.):

---

*Other medicines you are taking:*

*Doctor's name:*                              *Phone number:*

Source: "Teach Your Patients about Asthma," National Heart, Lung, and Blood Institute, October 1992.

# My Asthma Medicines

Ask your doctor the questions below. Write down what your doctor says for each medicine prescribed to you.

Name of medicine

_____

_____

When and how much you should take

_____

_____

How long to take it

_____

_____

What does the medicine do and when will I feel it working

_____

_____

_____

What to do if I forget to take it

_____

_____

_____

Side effects and what to do about them

_____

_____

_____

_____

When to call the doctor

_____

_____

_____

Source: "Your Asthma Can Be Controlled," National Heart, Lung, and Blood Institute, National Institutes of Health.

# Beta$_2$-agonists

## ACTION

Beta$_2$-agonists are bronchodilator medicines that open airways by relaxing the muscles in and around the airways that tighten during an asthma episode.

## HOW THEY ARE PRESCRIBED

Beta$_2$-agonists come in many forms. There are also many ways to take them. Beta$_2$-agonists can be:

- inhaled using a metered dose inhaler
- inhaled using a nebulizer
- a powder-filled capsule that is inhaled by using a device called a dry powder inhaler
- swallowed as a liquid or tablet
- taken as shots

Inhaled beta$_2$-agonists stop symptoms of asthma episodes and prevent asthma symptoms that are started by exercise. They are sometimes used in small doses (no more than three to four times a day) to keep daily asthma symptoms under control.

## SIDE EFFECTS

Side effects include rapid heartbeat, tremors, feeling anxious, and nausea. These side effects tend to leave as the body adjusts to the medicine. Serious side effects are rare, but may include chest pain, fast or irregular heartbeat, severe headache or feeling dizzy, very bad nausea, or vomiting. Call your doctor right away if you have any of these symptoms.

## NOTES

Inhaled medicines are the first choice. They begin to work within 5 minutes and have fewer side effects. The medicine goes right to the lungs and does not easily go into the rest of the body.

Liquids or tablets begin to work within 30 minutes and last as long as 4 to 6 hours.

A child as young as 5 years of age can use the metered dose inhaler. A holding chamber or spacer device (a tube attached to the inhaler) can be attached to the inhaler to make it easier to use and can help even younger children use a metered dose inhaler.

*continues*

continued

Using a nebulizer to take the medicine works the same way as using an inhaler. A nebulizer is easier to use than an inhaler. It is good for a child under age 5, for a patient who has trouble using an inhaler, or for a patient with *severe* asthma episodes.

Shots are sometimes used in a doctor's office or an emergency room for severe episodes. They work very fast but only last 20 minutes.

**REMEMBER Beta$_2$-agonists relieve symptoms, but they cannot reduce or prevent the swelling that causes the symptoms.** When you have to use a beta$_2$-agonist a lot, it may be a sign that the swelling in your airways is getting worse. If you use a beta$_2$-agonist to relieve symptoms every day or if you use it more than 3 or 4 times in a single day, your asthma may be getting much worse. You may need another kind of medicine, and you need to discuss this with your doctor right away.

**NOTES:**

Source: "Teach Your Patients about Asthma," National Heart, Lung, and Blood Institute, October 1992.

# Theophylline

## ACTION

Theophylline is a bronchodilator medicine that opens airways by relaxing the muscles in and around the airways that tighten during an asthma episode.

## HOW IT IS PRESCRIBED

Theophylline comes in three forms:

- tablets to be swallowed
- capsules to be swallowed
- liquid to be swallowed

Do not chew theophylline if taken in a tablet form, because too much of the time-released medicine will be released all at once.

If theophylline is taken in capsule form, you may open up the capsule and sprinkle it on a small amount of sweet, soft food such as yogurt, jelly, or honey to disguise the taste. Do not chew the capsule.

Do not mix theophylline with hot food. This will dissolve the medicine and release too much into the body.

Take theophylline with food rather than on an empty stomach.

If you forget to take your theophylline on time, do not take twice as much the next time. Take the normal amount as soon as you remember. Call your doctor about how to get back on schedule.

## SIDE EFFECTS

Side effects may include nausea, vomiting, stomach cramps, diarrhea, headache, muscle cramps, irregular heartbeat, and/or feeling shaky or restless. Call your doctor if you have any of these side effects. It may mean that the amount of medicine you are taking should be changed. Mild side effects often go away after a few days.

## NOTES

Theophylline may be prescribed to be taken every 8 or every 12 hours. This makes it an easy medicine to use.

*continues*

continued

It takes some time for theophylline to build up in the bloodstream, where it must stay at a constant amount to have a lasting effect. This means that it is important for you to take it at the time and in the amount that the doctor says.

Your doctor will do a simple blood test to see if the medicine is at the right level.

If your child has a fever or a virus (for example, chickenpox), or if your child starts taking an antibiotic, call your doctor right away. The usual dose may be too strong for your child during this time and your child may get sick from the theophylline.

Source: "Teach Your Patients about Asthma," National Heart, Lung, and Blood Institute, October 1992.

# Cromolyn

## ACTION

Cromolyn is an anti-inflammatory medicine that prevents airways from swelling when they come in contact with an asthma trigger.

## HOW IT IS PRESCRIBED

Cromolyn comes in three forms:

- a metered dose inhaler
- liquid that is used in a nebulizer
- a powder-filled capsule that is inhaled by using a device called a dry powder inhaler

Cromolyn can be used in two ways:

- To prevent symptoms of asthma, it should be taken every day.
- To prevent symptoms of asthma that occur with exercise or contact with an asthma trigger (such as an animal), it can be taken 5 to 60 minutes before contact. The effects of the medicine last for 3 or 4 hours.

## SIDE EFFECTS

Cromolyn is safe to use in the treatment of asthma. The only side effect is a dry cough. You can avoid this side effect by rinsing your mouth and drinking a few sips of water after taking it.

## NOTES

Cromolyn cannot be used to stop an asthma episode once it has started. Cromolyn can only be used to keep an episode from starting.

Cromolyn does not work for every patient. It may take up to 6 weeks for the medicine to take effect.

If you use an inhaled $beta_2$-agonist and cromolyn, take the $beta_2$-agonist first.

If you forget to take your cromolyn on time, take it as soon as you remember. Talk to your doctor about how to get back on your normal schedule.

Source: "Teach Your Patients about Asthma," National Heart, Lung, and Blood Institute, October 1992.

# Corticosteroids

## ACTION

Corticosteroids are anti-inflammatory medicines that prevent and reduce swelling inside the airways and decrease the amount of mucus in the lungs.

## HOW THEY ARE PRESCRIBED

Corticosteroids come in three forms:

- A metered dose inhaler
- Liquids or tablets to be swallowed (called oral corticosteroids)
- Shots

**Inhaled corticosteroids** are taken with a metered dose inhaler. When taken at the proper doses, they are safe medicines that work well for patients with moderate or severe asthma. They reduce the sensitivity of the airways to triggers, and they prevent swelling in the airways.

**Liquid and tablet (oral) corticosteroids** are used in serious asthma episodes to reduce swelling of the airways and prevent the episodes from getting even more severe. For people with moderate asthma, oral corticosteroids are sometimes used for 3 to 7 days and then stopped. People with very severe asthma may take oral corticosteroids every other morning or daily.

**Shots of corticosteroids** are used only in a doctor's office or emergency room for serious episodes.

## SIDE EFFECTS

Inhaled corticosteroids may cause a yeast infection in the mouth or bother the upper airways and cause coughing. There are two things to do to keep these things from taking place. Use a spacer device (an attachment on the inhaler) and rinse out your mouth after you take the medicine.

Using oral corticosteroids for a short time may cause different side effects. You may have a better appetite, fluid retention, weight gain, rounding of the face, changes in mood, and high blood pressure. These will stop when you quit taking the medicine, but **do not stop taking this medicine without first talking to your doctor.**

Oral corticosteroids used for a long time may have bad side effects such as high blood pressure, thinning of the bones, cataracts, muscle weakness, and slower growth in children. Because of these side effects, doctors should only use oral corticosteroids for a long time if a patient's asthma is serious.

*continues*

continued

## NOTES

Corticosteroids are not the same as the steroids used by some athletes. Inhaled corticosteroids and oral corticosteroids taken for a short time do not damage the liver and they do not cause other long-lasting changes in the body.

Children as young as 3 years of age can use inhaled corticosteroids if a holding chamber or spacer device is attached to the metered dose inhaler. Ask your doctor about this.

When oral corticosteroids are used to treat serious asthma episodes, they take about 3 hours to start working and are most effective in 6 to 12 hours.

Talk to your doctor about what to do when you forget to take your medicine on time.

## NOTES:

Source: "Teach Your Patients about Asthma," National Heart, Lung, and Blood Institute, October 1992.

# How To Use a Spray Inhaler

Remember to breathe in slowly.

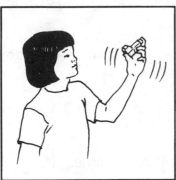

1. Take off the cap. Shake the inhaler.

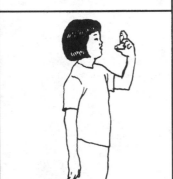

2. Stand up. Breathe out.

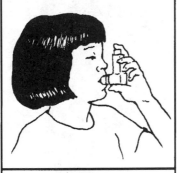

3. Put the inhaler in your mouth or put it just in front of your mouth. As you start to breathe in, push down on the top of the inhaler and keep breathing in slowly.

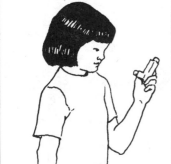

4. Hold your breath for 10 seconds. Breathe out.

*continues*

continued

## A spacer or a holding chamber makes it easier to use a spray inhaler.

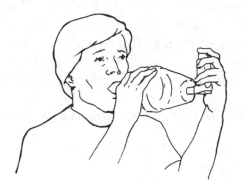

1. Spray the asthma medicine into the spacer one time.

2. Then take a deep breath and hold it for 10 seconds.

3. Breathe out into the spacer.

4. Breathe in again, but do not spray the medicine again.

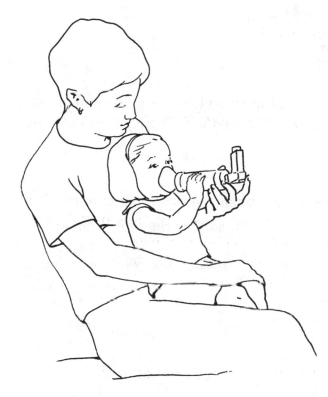

There are many kinds of spacers. Some have a mouthpiece. Some have a face mask.

Source: "Global Initiative for Asthma, What You and Your Family Can Do about Asthma," National Heart, Lung, and Blood Institute, December 1995.

# Your Metered-Dose Inhaler—How To Use It

Using a metered-dose inhaler is a good way to take asthma medicines. There are few side effects because the medicine goes right to the lungs and not to other parts of the body. It takes only 5 to 10 minutes for inhaled beta$_2$-agonists to have an effect compared to the liquid or pill form, which can take 15 minutes to 1 hour. Inhalers can be used by all asthma patients age 5 and older. A spacer or holding chamber attached to the inhaler can help make taking the medicine easier.

The inhaler must be cleaned often to prevent buildup that will clog it or reduce how well it works.

- The guidelines that follow will help you use the inhaler the correct way.
- Ask your doctor or nurse to show you how to use the inhaler.

## USING THE INHALER

1. Remove the cap and hold the inhaler upright.
2. Shake the inhaler.
3. Tilt your head back slightly and breathe out.
4. Use the inhaler in any one of these ways. (A and B are the best ways. B is recommended for young children, older adults, and those taking inhaled steroids. C is okay if you are having trouble with A or B.)

    A. Open mouth with inhaler 1 to 2 inches away.
    B. Use a spacer (ask for the handout on spacers).
    C. Put inhaler in mouth and seal lips around the mouthpiece.

5. Press down on the inhaler to release the medicine as you start to breathe in slowly.
6. Breathe in **slowly** for 3 to 5 seconds.
7. **Hold** your breath for 10 seconds to allow the medicine to reach deeply into your lungs.

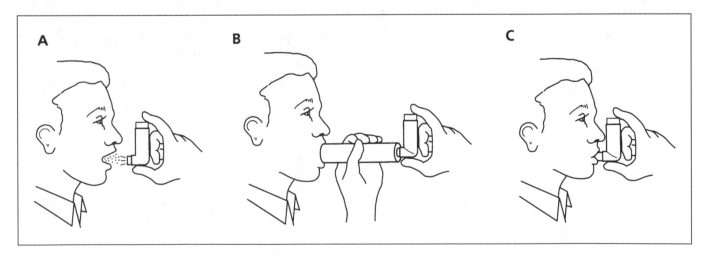

*continues*

continued

8. Repeat puffs as prescribed. Waiting 1 minute between puffs may permit the second puff to go deeper into the lungs.

Note: Dry powder capsules are used differently. To use a dry powder inhaler, close your mouth tightly around the mouthpiece and inhale very fast.

## CLEANING

1. Once a day clean the inhaler and cap by rinsing it in warm running water. Let it dry before you use it again. Have another inhaler to use while it is drying. Do not put the canister holding cromolyn or nedocromil in water.
2. Twice a week wash the L-shaped plastic mouthpiece with mild dishwashing soap and warm water. Rinse and dry well before putting the canister back inside the mouthpiece.

## CHECKING HOW LONG A CANISTER WILL LAST

1. Check the canister label to see how many "puffs" it contains.
2. Figure out how many puffs you will take per day (for example, 2 puffs, 4 times a day = 8 puffs a day). Divide this number into the number of puffs contained in the canister. That tells you how long the canister should last.

Example

Canister contains 200 puffs.
You take 2 puffs, 4 times a day, which equal 8 puffs/day.
200 ÷ 8 = 25. The canister will last 25 days.

Source: "Nurses: Partners in Asthma Care," National Asthma Education and Prevention Program, National Heart, Lung, and Blood Institute, NIH Publication No. 95-3308, 1995.

# Medicamentos inhalados para el asma

La mejor manera para la administración de medicamentos para tratar el asma es la inhalada. Se han introducido muchos aparatos diferentes en las últimas décadas para permitir a los asmáticos de todas las edades usar medicamentos inhalados para ayudarlos a controlar su problema respiratorio. Las principales ventajas de los medicamentos inhalados son: (1) su administración directa al punto causante del problema (los bronquios y bronquiolos que conducen a los pulmones) y (2) la falta de efectos secundarios relacionados a los medicamentos administrados por vía sistémica (usualmente por vía oral).

## TIPOS DE MEDICAMENTOS INHALADOS

Se encuentran disponibles en forma inhalada cuatro tipos de medicamentos para el asma:

1. Broncodilatadores beta$_2$ agonistas, que son los más comúnmente usados. Estos incluyen albuterol, bitolterol, pirbutero, y terbutalina, que se usan como medicamentos de "rescate" para aliviar los ataques de asma. Estos inhaladores pueden utilizarse en exceso, el uso de más de un frasco por mes resulta en motivo de preocupación. El salmeterol es un broncodilatador nuevo beta$_2$ agonista de larga acción que se usa como mantenimiento del control del asma.

2. El Ipratropium, es un broncodilatador anti-colinérgico.

3. Los corticoesteroides inhalados son medicamentos anti-inflamatorios potentes. Ejemplos son la beclometasona, budesonide (se espera que se apruebe pronto para su uso en los E.U.A.), flunisolida, fluticasona y triamcinolona.

4. Medicamentos anti-inflamatorios no-esteroideos como el cromoglicato y el nedocromil.

## TIPOS DE APARATOS PARA INHALACIÓN

Existen tres tipos básicos de aparatos usados para administrar medicamentos inhalados. El más común de estos es el inhalador de dosis medida (IDM). Todos los medicamentos mencionados se encuentran disponibles con IDM.

Los nebulizadores se emplean frecuentemente para lactantes asmáticos y niños pequeños y en pacientes con enfermedad aguda de todas las edades. Estos aparatos administran pequeñas gotas del medicamento usando oxígeno o aire bajo presión. Actualmente se encuentran disponibles para nebulización en los E.U.A. albuterol, ipratropium, cromoglicato, budesonide.

Se han utilizado inhaladores de rotación para administrar cromoglicato, y se usan actualmente para el albuterol inhalado. Un aparato similar ha sido probado en los E.U.A. para la inhalación del budesonide y estará disponible pronto. La mayor parte de los medicamentos inhalados para el asma se obtendrán en esta forma ya que el gobierno está preocupado acerca de los efectos

*continúa*

continuación

ambientales de los clorofluorcarbonos (CFC) usados como agentes impulsores en la mayoría de los IDM.

## ESPACIADORES Y CÁMARAS

Muchos de los niños pequeños y algunos adultos tienen problemas para coordinar la inhalación con el disparo de un inhalador de dosis medida (IDM). Estos pacientes pueden preferir usar un espaciador. Los estudios muestran que un porcentaje mayor del medicamento es depositado en las vías respiratorias más bajas, en lugar de la garganta, después del uso de un IDM con un espaciador de volumen grande. Aquellos con cámaras de apoyo y válvulas de una vía para prevenir que se escape el medicamento tienen la ventaja de permitir al asmático respirar más cerca de su ritmo mientras se encuentra inhalando dosis efectivas de medicamento. Por lo menos una versión de un espaciador de volumen grande con cámara y una válvula se encuentra disponible con una máscara que viene en tres tamaños para los lactantes, niños y adultos.

## SE NECESITA ENTRENAMIENTO ADECUADO

Todos los inhaladores de dosis medida (IDM) traen instrucciones. Es muy importante seguir estas instrucciones cuidadosamente. Los individuos asmáticos y/o sus encargados de cuidarlos deben solicitar al médico que los prescriba que les dé una demostración del uso del IDM específico que vaya a usarse. Esta deberá hacerse nuevamente en la farmacia si es necesario. Se deberá revisar la técnica en las visitas de control. Los tipos de IDM usados para administrar albuterol, beclometasona, cromoglicato, fluticasona, ipratropium, nedocromil, salmeterol y terbutalina son todos muy similares entre sí. Las siguientes instrucciones corresponden a todos estos inhaladores:

1. Agite bien el inhalador inmediatamente antes de cada uso.

2. Quite la tapa de la boquilla. Si no hay tapa, verifique la boquilla abriéndola para ver si no hay objetos extraños antes de cada uso.

3. Asegúrese de que el recipiente no se encuentre vacío recordando cuántas inhalaciones se han administrado. Un fabricante incluye un "verificador de atomizaciones" en las indicaciones del paciente. También existe en el mercado un aparato que el paciente puede insertar en su inhalador para registrar el número de inhalaciones aplicadas. Para los medicamentos de mantenimiento tomados a diario, puede dividir el número de inhalaciones por frasco (escritas en el recipiente y/o en la información del paciente que viene con el medicamento) por el número de atomizaciones diarias para calcular cuántos días va a durar y cuándo debe cambiar su IDM. El método de inmersión ampliamente usado es probablemente muy poco exacto para confiar en él.

4. Verifique el aerosol del inhalador antes de usarlo por primera vez o si no ha sido usado en más de cuatro semanas. (No necesita hacerlo después cada vez que lo vaya a usar).

5. Exhale por la boca para vaciar los pulmones.

*continúa*

continuación

6. Coloque la boquilla en la boca, dejando la lengua debajo. Como alternativa, el inhalador puede colocarse a 1 ó 2 pulgadas de distancia de la boca abierta.

7. Mientras inhala profundamente y despacio a través de la boca, presione hacia abajo con firmeza y completamente en la parte de arriba del frasco de metal con su dedo índice.

8. Continúe inhalando todo lo que pueda y trate de mantener la respiración por 5-10 segundos. Antes de respirar hacia afuera, quite el inhalador de la boca y quite el dedo del frasco.

9. Espere 30-60 segundos y agite el inhalador otra vez. Repita estos pasos en cada inhalación que le haya recetado su médico.

10. Coloque en su lugar la tapa de la boquilla después de cada uso.

11. Limpie el inhalador completamente y frecuentemente. Quite el bote de metal y limpie el estuche plástico y la tapa enjuagándolos con agua corriente caliente, por lo menos una vez al día. No sumerja frascos de metal que contengan cromoglicato y nedocromil. Después de secar completamente el estuche plástico y la tapa, ponga en su lugar con cuidado el frasco mediante un giro y coloque la tapa.

12. Deseche el bote después de que haya usado el número señalado de inhalaciones. No se puede estar seguro de la cantidad correcta de medicamento después de este punto.

**Nota:** Los IDM usados para la administración de bitolterol, pilbuterol y triamcinolona son de cierto modo diferentes de los otros. Es muy importante seguir las instrucciones específicas incluyendo las de estos inhaladores. Los espaciadores y cámaras de aire que se encuentran en el comercio también vienen con instrucciones que modifican de algún modo las instrucciones mencionadas. Para "estar seguro" obtenga el entrenamiento específico para cada uno de los inhaladores que le receten.

## USO DE NEBULIZADORES

Existen muchos nebulizadores en el mercado. Los más caros son los portátiles, con características como tamaño de peso ligero, paquetes de baterías y adaptadores para usar en automóviles. Pero aún los nebulizadores menos caros administran de un modo efectivo los medicamentos para el asma en gota fina, a través de máscaras de diferentes tamaños de lactantes hasta para adultos, a través de tubos-T o por adaptadores de boquilla. Los medicamentos nebulizados para el asma son especialmente útiles en lactantes, niños pequeños y algunos pacientes ancianos que no pueden usar un IDM, aún con una cámara de aire con máscara. Es también frecuentemente útil en niños mayores y adultos para ayudar a revertir una crisis de asma aguda.

Una vez más el entrenamiento adecuado es necesario. Este puede ser proporcionado por personal del consultorio o el médico que recetó el tratamiento nebulizado. Este entrenamiento es frecuentemente proporcionado por compañías de suministro médico que equipan los nebulizadores. Su personal irá a la casa del paciente a entregar el nebulizador y entrenarlo.

Courtesy of American Academy of Allergy, Asthma and Immunology, 1-800-822-2762, www.aaai.org.

# Spacers—Making Inhaled Medicines Easier To Take

Unless you use your inhaler the right way, much of the medicine may end up on your tongue, on the back of your throat, or in the air. Use of a spacer or holding chamber can help prevent this problem.

A spacer or holding chamber is a device that attaches to a metered-dose inhaler. It holds the medicine in its chamber long enough for you to inhale it in one or two slow deep breaths.

The spacer makes it easy to use the medicines the right way (especially if your child is young or you have a hard time using just an inhaler). It helps you not cough when using an inhaler. A spacer will also help prevent you from getting a yeast infection in your mouth (thrush) when taking inhaled steroid medicines.

There are many models of spacers or holding chambers that you can purchase through your pharmacist or a medical supply company. Ask your doctor about the different models.

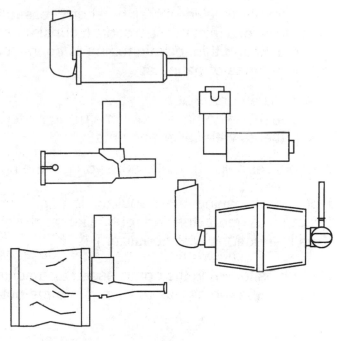

*There are a variety of spacers.*

## HOW TO USE A SPACER

1. Attach the inhaler to the spacer or holding chamber as explained by your doctor or by using the directions that come with the product.
2. Shake well.
3. Press the button on the inhaler. This will put one puff of the medicine in the holding chamber.
4. Place the mouthpiece of the spacer in your mouth, and inhale slowly. (A face mask may be helpful for a young child.)
5. Hold your breath for a few seconds and then exhale. Repeat steps 4 and 5.
6. If your doctor has prescribed two puffs, wait between puffs for the amount of time he or she has directed and repeat steps 2 through 5.

Source: "Nurses: Partners in Asthma Care," National Asthma Education and Prevention Program, National Heart, Lung, and Blood Institute, NIH Publication No. 95-3308, 1995.

# How To Use and Care for Your Nebulizer

A nebulizer is a device driven by a compressed air machine. It allows you to take asthma medicine in the form of a mist (wet aerosol). It consists of a cup, a mouthpiece attached to a T-shaped part or a mask, and thin, plastic tubing to connect to the compressed air machine. It is used mostly by three types of patients:

- children under age 5
- patients who have problems using metered-dose inhalers
- patients with severe asthma

A nebulizer helps to make sure you get the right amount of medicine.

Routinely cleaning the nebulizer is important because an unclean nebulizer may cause an infection. A good cleaning routine keeps the nebulizer from clogging up and helps it last longer. (See instructions with nebulizer.)

Directions for using the compressed air machine may vary (check the machine's directions), but generally the tubing has to be put into the outlet of the machine before it is turned on.

## HOW TO USE A NEBULIZER

1a. **If your medicine is premixed**, measure the correct amount of medicine using a clean dropper and put it into the cup. Go to step 2.
1b. **If the medicine is not premixed**, measure the correct amount of saline—using a clean dropper—and put it into the cup. Then measure the correct amount of medicine using a *different* clean dropper and put it into the cup with the saline. (Do NOT mix the droppers; use one for saline and another for the medicine.) Put an "S" for saline on one dropper with nail polish.
2. Fasten the mouthpiece to the T-shaped part and then fasten this unit to the cup **OR** fasten the mask to the cup. For a child over the age of 2, use a mouthpiece unit because it will deliver more medicine than a mask.
3. Put the mouthpiece in your mouth. Seal your lips tightly around it **OR** place the mask on your face.
4. Turn on the air compressor machine.
5. Take slow, deep breaths in through the mouth.
6. Hold each breath 1 to 2 seconds before breathing out.
7. Continue until the medicine is gone from the cup (approximately 10 minutes).
8. Store the medicine as directed after each use.

*continues*

continued

## CLEANING THE NEBULIZER

**Don't forget:** Cleaning and getting rid of germs prevent infection. Cleaning keeps the nebulizer from clogging up and helps it last longer.

### Cleaning Needed after Each Use

1. Remove the mask or the mouthpiece and T-shaped part from the cup. Remove the tubing and set it aside. The tubing should not be washed or rinsed. The outside should be wiped down. Rinse the mask or mouthpiece and T-shaped part—as well as the eyedropper or syringe—in warm running water for 30 seconds. Use distilled or sterile water for rinsing if possible.
2. Shake off excess water. Air dry on a clean cloth or paper towel.
3. Put the mask or the mouthpiece and T-shaped part, cup, and tubing back together and connect the device to the compressed air machine. Run the machine for 10 to 20 seconds to dry the inside of the nebulizer.
4. Disconnect the tubing from the compressed air machine. Store the nebulizer in a ziplock plastic bag.
5. Place a cover over the compressed air machine.

### Cleaning Needed Once Every Day

1. Remove the mask or the mouthpiece and T-shaped part from the cup. Remove the tubing and set it aside. The tubing should not be washed or rinsed.
2. Wash the mask or the mouthpiece and T-shaped part—as well as the eyedropper or syringe—with a mild dishwashing soap and warm water.
3. Rinse under a strong stream of water for 30 seconds. Use distilled (or sterile) water if possible.
4. Shake off excess water. Air dry on a clean cloth or paper towel.
5. Put the mask or the mouthpiece and T-shaped part, cup, and tubing back together, and connect the device to the compressed air machine. Run the machine for 10 to 20 seconds to dry the inside of the nebulizer.
6. Disconnect the tubing from the compressed air machine. Store the nebulizer in a resealable plastic bag.
7. Place a cover over the compressed air machine.

### Cleaning Needed Once or Twice a Week

1. Remove the mask or the mouthpiece and T-shaped part from the cup. Remove the tubing and set it aside. The tubing should not be washed or rinsed. Wash the mask or the mouth-

*continues*

continued

    piece and T-shaped part—as well as the eyedropper or syringe—with a mild dishwashing soap and warm water.

2. Rinse under a strong stream of water for 30 seconds.

3. Soak for 30 minutes in a solution that is one part distilled white vinegar and two parts distilled water. Throw out the vinegar water solution after use; do not reuse it.

4. Rinse the nebulizer parts and the eyedropper or syringe under warm running water for 1 minute. Use distilled or sterile water if possible.

5. Shake off excess water. Air dry on a clean cloth or paper towel.

6. Put the mask or the mouthpiece and T-shaped part, cup, and tubing back together, and connect the device to the compressed air machine. Run the machine for 10 to 20 seconds to dry the inside of the nebulizer thoroughly.

7. Disconnect the tubing from the compressed air machine. Store the nebulizer in a resealable plastic bag.

8. Clean the surface of the compressed air machine with a well-wrung, soapy cloth or sponge. You could also use an alcohol or disinfectant wipe. **NEVER PUT THE COMPRESSED AIR MACHINE IN WATER.**

9. Place a cover over the compressed air machine.

**NOTES:**

Source: "Nurses: Partners in Asthma Care," National Asthma Education and Prevention Program, National Heart, Lung, and Blood Institute, NIH Publication No. 95-3308, 1995.

# Warning Signs of Asthma Episodes

Asthma episodes rarely occur without warning. Most people with asthma have warning signs (physical changes) that occur hours before symptoms appear. Warning signs are not the same for everyone. You may have different signs at different times. By knowing your warning signs and acting on them, you may be able to avoid a serious episode of asthma.

- Think back on your last asthma episode. Did you have any of the signs below?
- Check *your* warning sign(s). Show them to your doctor and family.
- Remember to follow your asthma control plan as soon as these signs appear.

**CHECK HERE**

- ☐ Drop in peak flow reading
- ☐ Chronic cough, especially at night
- ☐ Difficulty breathing
- ☐ Chest starts to get tight or hurts
- ☐ Breathing faster than normal
- ☐ Getting out of breath easily
- ☐ Tired
- ☐ Itchy, watery, or glassy eyes
- ☐ Stroking chin or throat
- ☐ Sneezing
- ☐ Head stopped up
- ☐ Headache
- ☐ Fever
- ☐ Restless
- ☐ Runny nose
- ☐ Change in face color
- ☐ Dark circles under eyes
- ☐ Other: _____

My most common warning signs of an asthma episode are:

1. _____

2. _____

3. _____

Source: "Teach Your Patients about Asthma," National Heart, Lung, and Blood Institute, October 1992.

# What To Do for an Asthma Attack

**Act fast if an asthma attack starts**

- Know the signs that an asthma episode is starting.

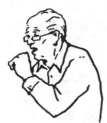 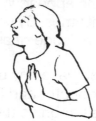 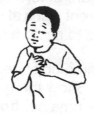 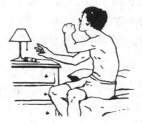

Cough          Wheeze          Tight chest          Wake up
                                                     at night

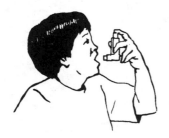

- Move away from the thing that started the attack.

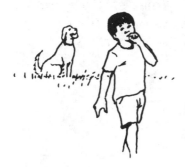

- Take a quick-relief asthma medicine.

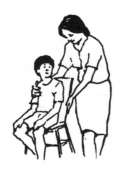

- Stay calm for 1 hour to be sure breathing gets better.

*continues*

continued

**Get emergency help from a doctor if you do not get better.**

Get immediate help if you see any of these asthma danger signs:

- Your quick-relief medicine does not help for very long or it does not help at all. Breathing is still fast and hard.
- It is hard to talk.
- Lips or fingernails turn grey or blue.
- The nose opens wide when the person breathes.
- Skin is pulled in around the ribs and neck when the person breathes.
- The heartbeat or pulse is very fast.
- It is hard to walk.

**Be careful! Using too much quick-relief medicine for asthma attacks can hurt you.**

Quick-relief medicine for asthma makes you feel better for a little while. It may stop the attack. With some attacks, you may think you are getting better but the airways are actually getting more and more swollen. Then you are in danger of having a very bad asthma attack that could kill you.

- If you use quick-relief medicine every single day to stop asthma attacks, this means you need a preventive medicine for asthma.
- If you need quick-relief medicine more than four times in 1 day to stop asthma attacks, **you need help from a doctor today.**

**NOTES:**

Source: "Global Initiative for Asthma, What You and Your Family Can Do about Asthma," National Heart, Lung, and Blood Institute, December 1995.

# Summary of Steps To Manage Asthma Episodes

- Know your warning signs and peak flow zones so you can begin treatment early.
- Take the correct amount of medicine at the times the doctor has stated. If the asthma control plan includes increased dosage or a second medicine to be used during episodes, take it as prescribed. **Always call your doctor if you need to take more medicine than the doctor ordered.**
- Remove yourself or the child from the trigger if you know what it is. Treatment does not work as well if the patient stays around the trigger.
- Keep calm and relaxed. Family members must stay calm and relaxed too.
- Rest.
- Observe yourself or the child by noting changes in body signs such as wheezing, coughing, trouble breathing, and posture. If you have a peak flow meter, measure peak flow number 5 to 10 minutes after each treatment to see if peak flow is improving.
- Review the list below for signs to seek emergency medical care for asthma. They include:
  —Your wheeze, cough, or shortness of breath gets worse, even after the medicine has been given and had time to work. Most inhaled bronchodilator medicines produce an effect within 5 to 10 minutes. Discuss the time your medicines take to work with your doctor.
  —Your peak flow number goes down, or does not improve after treatment with bronchodilators, or drops to 50 percent or less of personal best. Discuss this peak flow level with your doctor.
  —Your breathing gets difficult. Signs of this are:
    - your chest and neck are pulled or sucked in with each breath
    - you are hunching over
    - you are struggling to breathe
  —You have trouble walking or talking
  —You stop playing or working and cannot start again
  —Your lips or fingernails are gray or blue. If this happens, **Go to the Emergency Room Now!**
- Keep your important information for seeking emergency care handy.
- Call a family member, friend, or neighbor to help you if needed.
- Immediately call a clinic, doctor's office, or hospital for help if needed.

## Do Not

- Do not drink a lot of water. Just drink normal amounts.
- Do not breathe warm moist air from a shower.
- Do not rebreathe into a paper bag held over the nose.
- Do not use over-the-counter cold remedies without first calling the doctor.

Source: "Teach Your Patients about Asthma," National Heart, Lung, and Blood Institute, October 1992.

# Sample Patient Asthma Management Plan

**ASTHMA ACTION PLAN**

Name: _____    Issue Date _____

| | | PEAK FLOW | | TREATMENT |
|---|---|---|---|---|
| ❶ | BEST | = [    ] | ▷ | Continue regular treatment |
| ❷ | <80% | = [    ] | ▷ | Double dose of: _____ |
| ❸ | <60% | = [    ] | ▷ | Start prednisone & call your doctor |
| ❹ | <40% | = [    ] | ▷ | Call emergency doctor or Dial 911 for ambulance |

**SYMPTOMS**          **TREATMENT**

| | SYMPTOMS | | TREATMENT |
|---|---|---|---|
| ❶ | Asthma under control | ▷ | Continue regular treatment |
| ❷ | Waking with asthma at night | ▷ | Double dose of: _____ |
| ❸ | Increasing breathlessness or poor response to _____ | ▷ | Start prednisone & call your doctor |
| ❹ | Severe attack | ▷ | Call emergency doctor or Dial 911 for ambulance |

Contact Dr. _____    Tel. _____

Source: "Global Initiative for Asthma, What You and Your Family Can Do about Asthma," National Heart, Lung, and Blood Institute, December 1995.

# Write a Plan for Controlling Your Asthma

Ask your doctor what you should do in an emergency. Write the answers below.

What are the signs that tell me to seek care quickly?

_____

_____

_____

What should I do if my medicines do not seem to be working?

_____

_____

_____

Where should I go to get care quickly?

_____

_____

Should I call my doctor first or go to the emergency room?

_____

_____

_____

_____

What do I do if I have an asthma emergency very late at night?

_____

_____

_____

When I call, what information will my doctor want (my symptoms, what medicines I have taken, when I took them, and my peak flow rate)?

_____

_____

_____

_____

Source: "Your Asthma Can Be Controlled," National Heart, Lung, and Blood Institute, National Institutes of Health.

# Pocket-Size Asthma Action Plan

## ASTHMA ACTION PLAN

Name: _____     Issue Date _____

|  | | PEAK FLOW | | TREATMENT |
|---|---|---|---|---|
| ❶ | BEST = | | ⇨ | Continue regular treatment |
| ❷ | <80% = | | ⇨ | Double dose of:_____ |
| ❸ | <60% = | | ⇨ | Start prednisone & call Doctor |
| ❹ | <40% = | | ⇨ | Call emergency Dr. or Dial 911 for ambulance |

|  | SYMPTOMS | | TREATMENT |
|---|---|---|---|
| ❶ | Asthma under control | ⇨ | Continue regular treatment |
| ❷ | Waking with asthma at night | ⇨ | Double dose of |
| ❸ | Increasing breathlessness or poor response to | ⇨ | Start prednisone & ring your Doctor |
| ❹ | Severe attack | ⇨ | Call emergency Dr. or Dial 911 for ambulance |

Contact Dr. _____ Tel. _____

Note: The credit card sized asthma self-management plan system illustrated here has now been assessed in two clinical trials and has been introduced in several countries, including Australia, New Zealand, and the United Kingdom.

Source: "Asthma Management and Prevention," Publication No. 96-3659A, U.S. Department of Health and Human Services, National Heart, Lung, and Blood Institute, National Institutes of Health, December 1995.

# Plan for Staying Active—for Children

Even with asthma, you can play and take part in many activities—including sports—like other kids.

Many kids with asthma cough or wheeze when they exercise, run, or play hard. This does not have to happen. Your asthma medicine will help you be active without coughing or wheezing. Some kids keep asthma symptoms from starting if they take a certain asthma medicine right before they start their activity. Talk to your doctor about this.

It also helps you feel good while you are active if you do stretching exercises ("warm up" and "cool down") before *and* after your activity. Here is a plan to help you be active:

- List the things you do now to stay active.
- List the things you'd like to try.
- Check off things you'll do to be more active.

### PHYSICAL ACTIVITIES I DO NOW

- 
- 
- 
- 
- 

### PHYSICAL ACTIVITIES I'D LIKE TO TRY

- 
- 
- 
- 
- 

### TO BE ACTIVE I WILL

☐ Talk to my parent(s) about an activity I would like to do.
☐ Try the activity to see if I can do it without wheezing.
☐ Show my parent(s) how much I can do without wheezing.
☐ Talk to my parents and my doctor about taking medicine before I begin to exercise. This will keep asthma attacks or episodes from starting.
☐ Take a break from the activity if I feel I may start wheezing. Follow my asthma control plan.
☐ Talk to teachers and coaches about my asthma. Ask them to help me stay active.

Source: "Teach Your Patients about Asthma," National Heart, Lung, and Blood Institute, October 1992.

# How To Set Guidelines for Your Child's Activities

Parents often want to prevent their child from having asthma episodes by putting limits on what the child can do. Remember: the goal is to have a plan that lets the child do what he or she wants. This means not putting any limits on the child's activities.

The ideas in the list that follows may help you keep your child active and healthy:

1. Before setting any limits, look at what your child can already do. Try to help your child do more. Do not make up rules that might hold him or her back without good reason.
2. Base any limits you set on what has really happened with your child. Do not base it on what you think might happen or on what might be true for others with asthma. No child with asthma is the same. Each child has different levels of physical fitness and maturity. Aim toward setting fewer or no limits and letting your child have more responsibility.
3. Discuss the limits you think are right with your child. Try to agree on limits that both of you can accept.
4. Discuss disagreements or doubts with your doctor so that he or she can help decide if the rules are necessary for your child.
5. Practice and review with your child those things that can help to manage an asthma episode if he or she accidentally goes beyond his or her limits.
6. To help your child do more, find specific ways to protect him or her from those things that can trigger asthma. For example, if your child is allergic to animal dander and wants to visit a friend who has a dog, have your child take asthma medicine before the visit or have the friend come to your house. Your child should not touch the animal.

**Other suggestions:** _____

_____

_____

_____

Source: "Teach Your Patients about Asthma," National Heart, Lung, and Blood Institute, October 1992.

# Plan for Staying Active—for Adults

Many people with asthma have symptoms, especially coughing or wheezing, when they are physically active. This does not need to happen. An important treatment goal is for you to take part in the physical activity of your choice without having symptoms. Your regular asthma medicine should help you do this. Some people with asthma keep symptoms from starting by taking inhaled asthma medicines (beta$_2$-agonist or cromolyn) right before they start their activity. Talk to your doctor about this. Exercise is important for your health. Asthma should not keep you from being active.

Remember, over 67 athletes in the 1984 Olympics had asthma. Many won medals!

Here are some ideas to help you make a plan to be physically active:

- List the things you do now to stay active including household chores.
- List the things you would like to try.
- Check off things you will do to increase your activity level.

### PHYSICAL ACTIVITIES I DO NOW

- 
- 
- 
- 
- 

### PHYSICAL ACTIVITIES I'D LIKE TO TRY

- 
- 
- 
- 
- 

### TO BE ACTIVE I WILL

- ☐ Choose one of the activities I'd like to try to see if I can do it without symptoms.
- ☐ Check my peak flow number before, during, and after the activity—did it go down?
- ☐ Take a break if I feel symptoms coming on—and follow my asthma control plan.
- ☐ Talk to my doctor about taking medicine before starting an activity in order to prevent asthma episodes.
- ☐ Talk to relatives, friends, and coworkers about my asthma. Ask them to help me stay active.

Source: "Teach Your Patients about Asthma," National Heart, Lung, and Blood Institute, October 1992.

# Clues for Deciding To Go to School or Work

You can probably go to school or work if you have any of these symptoms:

- Stuffy nose, but no wheezing

- A little wheezing that goes away after taking medicine

- Able to do usual daily activities

- No extra effort needed to breathe

- Peak flow number in the Green Zone

## CLUES FOR DECIDING TO STAY HOME FROM SCHOOL OR WORK

You should probably stay home if you have any of these symptoms:

- Infection, sore throat, or swollen, painful neck glands

- Fever over 100°F orally or 101°F rectally; face hot and flushed

- Wheezing or coughing that still bothers you 1 hour after taking the medicine

- Weakness or tiredness that makes it hard to take part in usual daily activities

- Breathing with difficulty or breathing very fast

- Peak flow below 65–70 percent of personal best number and no response to treatment

Source: "Teach Your Patients about Asthma," National Heart, Lung, and Blood Institute, October 1992.

# Helping Students Control Their Asthma

Getting control of asthma means recognizing asthma triggers (the factors that make asthma worse or cause an asthma episode), avoiding or controlling these triggers, following an asthma management plan, and having convenient access to asthma medications. It also means modifying physical activities to match the students' current asthma status.

## RECOGNIZE ASTHMA TRIGGERS

Each student with asthma has a list of triggers that can make his or her condition worse—that is, that increase airway inflammation and/or make the airways constrict, which makes breathing difficult. "Asthma Triggers" lists the most common triggers.

### Asthma Triggers

- **Exercise:** running or playing hard, especially in cold weather
- **Upper respiratory infections:** colds or flu
- **Laughing or crying hard**
- **Allergens**
  —Pollens: from trees, plants, and grasses, including freshly cut grass
  —Animal dander: from pets with fur or feathers
  —Dust and dust mites: in carpeting, pillows, and upholstery
  —Cockroach droppings
  —Molds
- **Irritants**
  —Cold air
  —Strong smells and chemical sprays, including perfumes, paint and cleaning solutions, chalk dust, lawn and turf treatments
  —Weather changes
  —Cigarette and other tobacco smoke

## AVOID OR CONTROL ASTHMA TRIGGERS

Some asthma triggers—like pets with fur or feathers—can be avoided. Others—like physical exercise—are important for good health and should be controlled rather than avoided.

### Actions To Consider

- Identify students' known asthma triggers and eliminate as many as possible. For example, keep animals with fur out of the classroom. Consult the students' asthma management plans for guidance.
- Use wood, tile, or vinyl floor coverings instead of carpeting.

*continues*

continued

- Schedule maintenance or pest control that involves strong irritants and odors for times when students are not in the area and the area can be well ventilated.
- Adjust schedules for students whose asthma is worsened by pollen or cold air. A midday or indoor physical education class may allow more active participation.
- Help students follow their asthma management plans. These plans are designed to keep asthma under control.

## FOLLOW THE ASTHMA MANAGEMENT PLAN

A student's asthma management plan is developed by the student, parent/guardian, and health care provider. Depending on the student's needs, the plan may be a brief information card or a more extensive individualized health plan (IHP). "Asthma Management Plan Contents" lists what asthma plans typically contain. A copy of the plan should be on file in the school office or health services office, with additional copies for the student's teachers and coaches. The plan—as well as the student's asthma medications—should be easily available for all on- and off-site activities before, during, and after school.

### Asthma Management Plan Contents

- Brief history of the student's asthma
- Asthma symptoms
- Information on how to contact the student's health care provider, parent/guardian
- Physician and parent/guardian signature
- List of factors that make the student's asthma worse
- The student's personal best peak flow reading if the student uses peak flow monitoring
- List of the student's asthma medications
- A description of the student's treatment plan, based on symptoms or peak flow readings, including recommended actions for school personnel to help handle asthma episodes

Supporting and encouraging each student's efforts to follow his or her asthma management plan is essential for the student's active participation in physical activities. Students with asthma need understanding from both teachers and students in dealing with their asthma. If students with asthma are teased about their condition, they may be embarrassed, avoid using their medication, or cut class. If students with asthma are encouraged to "tough it out," they may risk health problems or just give up.

### Actions To Consider

- Get a copy of each student's asthma management plan. Review the plan to identify the role of the teacher and coach in the student's asthma management plan.

*continues*

continued

- Teach asthma awareness and peer sensitivity. Use the activities in the Asthma Awareness curriculum to teach K-6 students about asthma. As students learn more about asthma, they can more easily offer support instead of barriers to their classmates with asthma.

## ENSURE THAT STUDENTS WITH ASTHMA HAVE CONVENIENT ACCESS TO THEIR MEDICATIONS

Many students with asthma require two different medications: one for daily control and prevention, the other to treat and relieve symptoms. These medications are usually taken by metered-dose inhaler. Preventive asthma medications are taken daily and usually can be scheduled for before and after school hours. However, some students may need to take preventive daily medication during school hours. All students with asthma need to have their medication that relieves symptoms available at school in case of unexpected exposure to asthma triggers, or an asthma episode. In addition, students with asthma often benefit from using their inhaled medication 5–10 minutes before exercise. If accessing the medication is difficult, inconvenient, or embarrassing, the student may be discouraged and fail to use the inhaler as needed. The student's asthma may become unnecessarily worse and his or her activities needlessly limited.

### Actions To Consider

- Provide students with asthma convenient access to their medications for all on- and off-site activities before, during, and after school. These medications prevent as well as treat symptoms and enable the student to participate safely and vigorously in physical activities.
- Enable students to carry and administer their own medications if the parent/guardian, health care provider, and school nurse so advise.

## MODIFY PHYSICAL ACTIVITIES TO MATCH CURRENT ASTHMA STATUS

Students who follow their asthma management plans and keep their asthma under control can usually participate vigorously in the full range of sports and physical activities. Activities that are more intense and sustained—such as long periods of running, basketball, and soccer—are more likely to provoke asthma symptoms or an asthma episode. However, Olympic medalists with serious asthma have demonstrated that these activities are possible with good asthma management.

When a student experiences asthma symptoms, or is recovering from a recent asthma episode, exercise should be temporarily modified in type, length, and/or frequency to help reduce the risk of further symptoms. The student also needs convenient access to his or her medications.

*continues*

continued

## Actions To Consider

- Include adequate warmup and cool-down periods. These help prevent or lessen episodes of exercise-induced asthma.

- Consult the student's asthma management plan, parent/guardian, or health care provider on the type and length of any limitations. Assess the student and school resources to determine how the student can participate most fully.

- Remember that a student who experiences symptoms or who has just recovered from an asthma episode is at even greater risk for additional asthma problems. Take extra care. Observe for asthma symptoms, and check the student's peak flow if he or she uses a peak flow meter. Review the student's asthma management plan if there are any questions.

- Monitor the environment for potential allergens and irritants, for example, a recently mowed field or refinished gym floor. If an allergen or irritant is present, consider a temporary change in location.

- Make exercise modifications as necessary to get appropriate levels of participation. For example, if running is scheduled, the student could walk the whole distance, run part of the distance, or alternate running and walking.

- Keep the student involved when any temporary but major modification is required. Ask the student to act, for example, as a scorekeeper, timer, or equipment handler until he or she can return to full participation. Dressing for a physical education class and participating at any level is better than being left out or left behind.

## RECOGNIZING SYMPTOMS AND TAKING APPROPRIATE ACTION

Recognizing asthma symptoms and taking appropriate action in response to the symptoms is crucial to asthma treatment and control.

### Symptoms That Require Prompt Action

Acute symptoms require prompt action to help students resume their activities as soon as possible. Prompt action is also required to prevent an episode from becoming more serious or even life threatening. "Acute Symptoms Requiring Prompt Action" lists the symptoms that indicate an acute asthma episode and the need for immediate action. The student's asthma plan and the school's emergency plan should be easily accessible so that all staff, substitutes, volunteers, and aides know what to do.

Symptoms of exercise-induced asthma (coughing, wheezing, pain, or chest tightness) may last several minutes to an hour or more. These symptoms are quite different from breathlessness (deep, rapid breathing) that quickly returns to normal after aerobic exercise.

*continues*

continued

---

### Acute Symptoms Requiring Prompt Action

- Coughing or wheezing
- Difficulty in breathing
- Chest tightness or pressure reported by the student
- Other signs, such as low peak flow readings as indicated on the asthma management plan

---

*Actions to Take*

- Stop the student's current activity.
- Follow the student's asthma management/action plan.
- Help the student use his or her inhaled medication.
- Observe for effect.
- **Get Emergency Help**
  1. **If the student fails to improve.**
  2. **If any of the symptoms listed on the student's asthma plan as emergency indicators are present.**
  3. **If any of the following symptoms are present (consider calling 911):**
     — The student is hunched over, with shoulders lifted, and straining to breathe.
     — The student has difficulty completing a sentence without pausing for breath.
     — The student's lips or fingernails turn blue.

### Signs That May Indicate Poorly Controlled Asthma

Students may have symptoms that do not indicate an acute episode needing immediate treatment, but instead indicate that their asthma is not under complete control.

---

### Signs That May Indicate Poorly Controlled Asthma

- A persistent cough
- Coughing, wheezing, chest tightness, or shortness of breath after vigorous physical activity, on a recurring basis
- Low level of stamina during physical activity or reluctance to participate.

---

The teachers and coaches who supervise students' physical activities are in a unique position to notice signs that a child who struggles with physical activity might in fact have asthma. Because

*continues*

continued

exercise provokes symptoms in most children with poorly controlled asthma, the student may need to be evaluated by his or her health care provider. It may also be that the student simply needs to follow his or her asthma management plan more carefully.

*Actions To Consider*

- Share observations of the symptoms with the school nurse and the student's parents or guardians. Helping students get the medical attention they need is an important way to help children become active and take control of their condition.
- Provide students convenient access to their asthma medication.

**Confusing Signs: Is It an Asthma Episode or a Need for More Support?**

At some times teachers and coaches may wonder if a student's reported symptoms indicate a desire for attention or a desire not to participate in an activity. At other times it may seem that students are overreacting to minimal symptoms.

It is always essential to respect the student's report of his or her own condition. If a student regularly asks to be excused from recess or avoids physical activity, a real physical problem may be present. It also may be that the student needs more assistance and support from his or her teacher and coach in order to become an active participant.

*Actions To Consider*

- Talk with the student to:
  —learn his or her concerns about asthma and activity
  —offer reassurance that you understand the importance of appropriate modifications or activity limits
  —develop a shared understanding about the conditions that require activity modifications or medications
- Consult with the school nurse, parent/guardian, or health care provider to find ways to ensure that the student is safe, feels safe, and is encouraged to participate actively.
- If the student uses a peak flow meter, remind him or her to use it. This may help the student appreciate his or her asthma status and appropriate levels of activity.

Source: "Asthma and Physical Activity in the School," NIH Publication No. 95-3651, U.S. Department of Health and Human Services, National Institutes of Health, September 1995.

# If You Have Asthma and You Are Pregnant

### THINGS TO KNOW

- Asthma symptoms will become worse for about one-third of pregnant women.
- Asthma symptoms may be most severe between 29 and 36 weeks of pregnancy.
- Asthma that is not under control may affect the health of your baby as well as your own health.

### WHAT TO DO

- Tell your doctor, nurse, or nurse midwife that you have asthma.
- Make regular visits to your doctor, nurse, or nurse midwife for asthma and for care of your unborn baby.
- Discuss with your doctor the medicines you take for asthma to make sure they will not affect your baby.
- Follow your asthma medicine plan. Most medicines for asthma are safe to take when you are pregnant if you follow your doctor's advice. **Remember: if your asthma is not under control, your lungs are not getting enough oxygen to your baby. Not giving the baby oxygen is a far greater risk than taking asthma medicines.**
- Try not to take these asthma-allergy medicines while you are pregnant:
  - **Decongestants.** These are medicines that break up or decrease excess mucus. Cold medicines often contain this type of medicine.
  - **Certain antibiotics** such as tetracycline.
  - **Live virus vaccine.** *Killed* virus vaccines are all right.

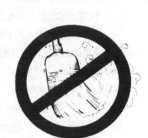

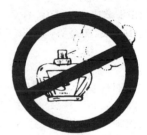

  - **Allergy Shots.** Do not begin allergy shots (but they may be continued if you were getting them before this pregnancy).
  - **Iodides.**
  - Medicines such as **brompheniramine, epinephrine, phenylephrine,** and **phenylpropanolamine.** Ask your doctor about these.

*continues*

continued

- Review and improve all actions you take to avoid or reduce contact with triggers of asthma. These triggers may include:
  —Tobacco smoke
  —House-dust mites
  —Animal dander
  —Pollen
  —Mold spores
  —Strong odors (for example, paint, perfume, and cooking)
  —Any other known allergen or irritant

## DON'T WORRY

- Wheezing during labor and delivery is rare.
- Most asthma medicines will not harm your baby. **REMEMBER: The best way to help your baby is to take care of your asthma.**
- Asthma medicines will not cause problems for your baby if you decide to breast feed.

**NOTES:**

Source: "Teach Your Patients about Asthma," National Heart, Lung, and Blood Institute, October 1992.

# If You Have Asthma and You Are Over Age 55

## WHAT TO DO

- Have a complete checkup to find out what other health problems you may have that could affect or be affected by your asthma. For example, asthma can affect heart disease. Theophylline can make high blood pressure worse.
- Discuss with your doctor the medicines you take for asthma and make sure they will not affect other health problems.
- Make regular visits to your doctor to check your asthma and any other health problems you may have.
- Discuss with your doctor any symptoms that you may have even if you don't think they are related to asthma.
- Report any physical problems you may have that might make it hard for you to take your asthma medicine.
  - If you have hearing problems and don't hear or understand the doctor or nurse, be sure to ask them to speak up. Ask questions. Be sure you understand what they want you to do.
  - If you have arthritis, a holding chamber or spacer device (a tube to attach to the inhaler) can make it easier to use a metered dose inhaler.
  - If you have vision problems, remember to wear your glasses when measuring medicines or peak flow numbers. **Ask for asthma handouts in larger type.**
  - If you have memory problems, ask the doctor to make your medicine plan as simple as possible to follow. **Be sure the plan is *written* down.**
- Get help from a support group, close friends or family members, or a counselor when you feel under great stress or are depressed. Changes in your life, like the death of a loved one or loss of a job, may cause these feelings. Although it is very rare, these problems may increase your chances of having an asthma episode that could threaten your life. You must take care of yourself to keep your asthma under control.
- If you are taking long-term steroid medicines, have regular checkups. Ask your doctor to check:
  - the number of your blood cells, your blood sugar, and your potassium
  - your eyes each year to be sure you are not getting cataracts or glaucoma
  - the health of your bones

Source: "Teach Your Patients about Asthma," National Heart, Lung, and Blood Institute, October 1992.

# If Your Infant Has Asthma, You Will Have To Take Extra Care

The lungs of a baby do not function as efficiently as the lungs of an older child. As a result, a severe episode of asthma can quickly result in lung failure.

## WHAT TO DO

- Follow the appointment schedule for checking on your baby's asthma. The doctor will want to see your child regularly even if he or she is not having symptoms.
- If your baby has asthma symptoms, act quickly. Follow the asthma control plan your doctor made for handling symptoms.
- Watch your baby closely for signs to seek emergency care. These signs include:
  —breathing rate increases (to over 40 breaths per minute while the infant is sleeping). Count the number of breaths in 15 seconds and multiply by four.
  —suckling or feeding stops
  —skin between the infant's ribs is pulled tight
  —chest gets bigger
  —coloring changes (pale or red face; fingernails turn blue)
  —cry changes in quality—becomes softer and shorter
  —nostrils open wider (nasal flaring)
  —grunting
- Be prepared. Do not wait until the last minute to learn how to handle an emergency. Have an asthma control plan to get to the doctor or hospital that includes knowing *how you'll get there, how much it will cost,* and *who will watch your other children*.

## DO NOT

During an asthma episode

- **Do not** give your baby large volumes of liquids to drink; just give normal amounts.
- **Do not** have your baby breathe warm, moist air (for example, the mist from a hot shower).
- **Do not** have your baby rebreathe into a bag held tightly over his or her nose and mouth.
- **Do not** give your baby over-the-counter antihistamines and cold medicines.

Source: "Teach Your Patients about Asthma," National Heart, Lung, and Blood Institute, October 1992.

# Occupational Asthma

Occupational asthma is a respiratory disorder directly related to inhaling fumes, gases, vapors or dust while "on the job." Due to this exposure, asthma may develop for the first time in a previously healthy worker, or pre-existing asthma may be aggravated. Symptoms of asthma include wheezing, chest tightness, and cough. Other associated symptoms may include runny nose, nasal congestion, and eye irritation. The cause may be allergic or non-allergic in nature. One notable symptom of occupational exposure is that the disease may persist for a lengthy period in some workers, even if they are no longer exposed to the irritants that caused it. Many workers with persistent asthma symptoms have been incorrectly diagnosed as having bronchitis.

It's important to remember that persons living in residential areas near these factories are often also exposed to these fumes and may suffer symptoms as well.

In many cases, a previous family history of allergy will make a person more likely to suffer from occupational asthma. However, many individuals who have no such history will still develop this disease if exposed to conditions that trigger it. Workers who smoke are at greater risk for developing asthma following some occupational exposures. The length of occupational exposure that triggers asthma varies and can range from months to years before symptoms occur.

## PREVALENCE

Occupational asthma has become the most prevalent work-related lung disease in developed countries. However, the exact proportion of newly diagnosed cases of asthma in adults due to occupational exposure is unknown. Researchers estimate that 15% of all male cases of asthma in Japan result from exposure to industrial vapors, dust, gases, or fumes, and up to 15% of asthma cases in the U.S. may have job-related origins.

The incidence of occupational asthma varies within individual industries. For example, in the detergent industry, inhalation of a particular enzyme used to produce washing powders has led to the development of respiratory symptoms in approximately 25% of exposed employees. In the printing profession, 20–50% of employees experience respiratory symptoms due to gum acacia, which is used in color printing to separate printed sheets and prevent smearing. Isocyanates are chemicals that are widely used in many industries, including spray painting, insulation installation, and in manufacturing plastics, rubber, and foam. These chemicals can lead to asthma in 10% of exposed workers.

## CAUSES

Occupational asthma may be caused by direct irritants, allergic triggers, or pharmacologic factors.

*continues*

continued

Irritants that provoke occupational asthma include exposure to hydrochloric acid, sulfur dioxide, or ammonia found in the petroleum or chemical industries. These asthmatic episodes frequently occur immediately after exposure to the substance, and allergic sensitization is not involved. Workers who already have asthma or some other respiratory disorder are particularly affected by this type of exposure.

Allergic factors play a role in many cases of occupational asthma. This type of asthma frequently requires long-term exposure to a work-related substance before allergic sensitization occurs. Examples of this allergic-type of occupational asthma include exposure to the enzymes of the bacteria bacillus subtilis in the washing powder industry, and exposure to castor beans, green coffee beans, and papain in the food processing industry. Other allergic forms of occupational asthma can occur in workers in the plastic, rubber, or resin industries following exposure to small chemical molecules in the air. Furthermore, veterinarians, fishermen, and animal handlers in laboratories can develop allergic reactions to animal proteins. Health care workers can develop asthma from aerosolized proteins from latex gloves or from the mixing of powdered medications.

Pharmacologic factors include the inhalation of dust or liquid. These substances do not lead to allergic sensitization, but instead directly lead to the release of naturally occurring substances such as histamine within the lung, which then in turn lead to asthma.

## PREVENTION

Once the cause is identified, exposure levels should be reduced (a worker could be moved to another job within the plant, for example).

Employers might consider pre-screening potential employees with lung function tests and then continue to test for symptoms after certain periods on the job once the worker has been hired.

Work areas should be closely monitored so that exposure to asthma-causing substances is kept at the lowest possible levels.

Under an allergist's care, pre-treatment with specific medications to counteract the effects of these substances may be helpful in some cases.

*continues*

continued

## COMMON AGENTS THAT CAUSE OCCUPATIONAL ASTHMA

| Agent | Workers At Risk |
|---|---|
| Acylate | Adhesives handlers |
| Amines | Shellac and lacquer handlers, solderers |
| Anhydrides | Users of plastics, epoxy resins |
| Animal-derived allergens | Animal handlers |
| Cereals | Bakers, millers |
| Chloramine-T | Janitors, cleaning staff |
| Drugs | Pharmaceutical workers, health professionals |
| Dyes | Textile workers |
| Enzymes | Detergent users, pharmaceutical workers, bakers |
| Fluxes | Electronic workers |
| Formaldehyde, glutaradehyde | Hospital staff |
| Gums | Carpet makers, pharmaceutical workers |
| Isocyanates | Spray painters, insulation installers, manufacturers of plastics, rubber & foam |
| Latex | Health professionals |
| Metals | Solderers, refiners |
| Persulfate | Hairdressers |
| Seafood | Seafood processors |
| Wood dusts | Forest workers, carpenters, cabinetmakers |

Courtesy of American Academy of Allergy, Asthma, and Immunology, 1-800-822-2762, www.aaaai.org.

# Asma ocupacional

El asma ocupacional se define como una enfermedad respiratoria directamente relacionada con la inhalación de emanaciones, gases o polvo "en el trabajo." El asma se puede presentar por primera vez en un trabajador previamente sano o el asma preexistente puede agravarse por la exposición en el sitio de trabajo. Los síntomas de asma incluyen resuello, opresión del pecho y tos. Otros síntomas asociados pueden incluir catarro, congestión nasal e irritación de ojos. La causa puede ser de índole alérgica o no alérgica. De particular importancia es el hecho de que la enfermedad puede persistir por un período largo en algunos trabajadores, aún cuando ya no se esté expuesto a los irritantes que la ocasionaron. Muchos trabajadores con síntomas persistentes de asma han sido mal diagnosticados como enfermos de bronquitis.

Es importante recordar que las personas que viven en áreas residenciales cerca de estas fábricas también pueden exponerse a estas emanaciones y llegar a presentar síntomas.

En muchos casos, los antecedentes familiares de alergia harán que una persona se encuentre más predispuesta a padecer asma ocupacional. Sin embargo, muchas personas sin estos antecedentes desarrollan la enfermedad si se exponen a condiciones que la desencadenen. Los trabajadores que fuman se encuentran en gran riesgo de desarrollar asma después de algunas exposiciones ocupacionales. La duración de la exposición ocupacional que desencadena el asma varía, pudiendo fluctuar entre meses y años antes de que se presenten los síntomas.

## FRECUENCIA

El asma ocupacional se ha convertido en la enfermedad pulmonar relacionada con el trabajo más prevaleciente en los países desarrollados. Sin embargo, se desconoce la proporción exacta de los casos nuevos diagnosticados de asma en adultos, debido a la exposición ocupacional. Los investigadores estiman que el 15% de todos los casos masculinos de asma en el Japón son el resultado de la exposición a vapores industriales, polvo, gases o emanaciones; además, del 5 la 15% de casos de asma en los E.U.A. podrían tener orígenes relacionados con el trabajo.

La incidencia de asma ocupacional varía dentro de cada industria. Por ejemplo, en la industria de detergentes, la inhalación de una enzima especial usada para producir detergentes en polvo ha contribuido a desarrollar síntomas respiratorios en aproximadamente el 25% de los empleados expuestos. En las imprentas, del 20 al 50% de los empleados presenta síntomas respiratorios debido a la goma acacia, la cual se usa en la impresión de color para separar hojas impresas y prevenir manchas. Los isocianatos son agentes químicos ampliamente usados en varias industrias, incluyendo pinturas en aerosol, instalaciones para aislamiento y en la fabricación de plásticos, caucho y espuma. Estos agentes químicos pueden llegar a inducir el asma en un 10% de los trabajadores expuestos.

*continúa*

continuación

# LAS CAUSAS

El asma ocupacional puede ser causada por uno de los tres mecanismos, incluyendo irritantes directos, desencadenantes alérgicos o factores farmacológicos. Los irritantes que provocan casos de asma ocupacional incluyen la exposición al ácido clorhídrico bióxido de sulfuro o amoníaco que se encuentra en industrias petroleras o químicas. Estos episodios asmáticos frecuentemente ocurren inmediatamente después de ocurrida la exposición a la sustancia irritante, y no implica la sensibilización alérgica. Los trabajadores que ya tengan asma, u otra enfermedad respiratoria, se ven especialmente afectados por este tipo de exposición.

Los factores alérgicos influyen en numerosos casos de asma ocupacional. Este tipo de asma frecuentemente requiere una exposición prolongada a una sustancia relacionada con el trabajo antes de que ocurra la sensibilización alérgica. Entre los ejemplos de este asma ocupacional de tipo alérgico se incluyen la exposición a las enzimas de la bacteria Bacillus subtilis, en la industria de detergentes en polvo; además de la exposición a las semillas de ricino, granos verdes de café y papaína en la industria procesadora de alimentos. Otras formas alérgicas de asma ocupacional pueden presentarse en trabajadores de las industrias de plásticos, caucho o resinas después de la exposición a moléculas químicas pequeñas en el aire. Además, los veterinarios, pescadores y manipuladores de animales en laboratorio pueden desarrollar reacciones alérgicas a las proteínas animales. Los trabajadores de la salud pueden desarrollar asma por las proteínas en aerosol de los guantes de látex o por la mezcla de medicamentos en polvo.

Los factores farmacológicos incluyen la inhalación de polvo o líquido. Estas sustancias no ocasionan la sensibilización alérgica, pero inducen a la liberación de sustancias naturales como la histamina dentro del pulmón, las cuales a su vez inducen al asma.

# PREVENCIÓN

1. Una vez identificada la causa, los niveles de exposición deben ser reducidos (por ejemplo un trabajador puede ser cambiado a otro trabajo dentro de la planta);
2. Los empleadores podrían considerar la preselección de trabajadores potenciales, exámenes de función pulmonar y continuar haciendo pruebas periódicamente en el trabajo una vez que el trabajador ya ha sido contratado;
3. Las áreas de trabajo deben ser cuidadosamente controladas para mantener al mínimo los niveles de la exposición a sustancias que causan asma;
4. Bajo el cuidado de un especialista en alergias, podría ser útil el pre-tratamiento con medicamentos específicos para contrarrestar los efectos de estas sustancias en algunos casos.

*continúa*

continuación

## AGENTES COMUNES QUE CAUSAN ASMA OCUPACIONAL

| Agentes | Trabajadores con riesgo potencial |
|---|---|
| Acrilato | Manipuladores de adhesivos |
| Alérgenos derivados de animales | Manipuladores de animales |
| Aminas | Soldadores, operadores de barniz y laca |
| Anhídridos | Usuarios de plásticos y resinas epóxidas |
| Cereales | Panaderos, molineros |
| Cloramina-T | Porteros, personal de aseo |
| Enzimas | Usuarios de detergentes, trabajadores farmacéuticos, paraderos |
| Fármacos | Trabajadores farmaceúticos, profesionales de la salud |
| Formaldehído, glutaraldehído | Personal de hospital |
| Gomas | Fabricantes de alfombras, trabajadores farmacéuticos |
| Isocianatos | Pintores con aerosoles, instaladores de aislantes |
| | Fabricantes de plásticos, caucho y espuma |
| Látex | Profesionales de la salud |
| Mariscos y pescados | Procesadores de mariscos y pescados |
| Metales | Soldadores, refinadores |
| Persulfato | Peluqueros |
| Polvo de madera | Trabajadores forestales, carpinteros, fabricantes especializados en ebanistería |
| Soldaduras | Trabajadores del área electrónica |
| Tintes | Trabajadores textiles |

Courtesy of American Academy of Allergy, Asthma, and Immunology, 1-800-822-2762, www.aaaai.org.

# Exercise-Induced Asthma and Bronchospasm

Most asthmatics have symptoms of wheezing during or following exercise. In addition, many non-asthmatic patients with allergies or a family history of allergy experience bronchospasm or constricted airways caused by exercise. Other symptoms include an accelerated heart rate, coughing, and chest tightness occurring five to ten minutes after exercise. The following can worsen symptoms:

- Exposure to cold air and low humidity, which increase heat loss from the airways;
- Nasal blockage, which prevents air from being humidified and warmed in the nose;
- Air pollutants, such as sulfur dioxide, high pollen counts, viral respiratory tract infections, and hot muggy air.

### Activities Most Likely To Cause Wheezing (in Order of Severity)

- Free running (most likely to induce asthma)
- Treadmill running
- Bicycling

### Testing Procedures

- The asthma specialist takes a patient history of wheezing and other asthmatic symptoms.
- A breathing test is done while the patient is at rest to see if the patient has undiagnosed asthma. This test may be repeated after exercise.
- Specialized tests, which can include cycling, running, or treadmill tests, are performed.

### TREATMENT

1. Carefully select exercise activities such as walking, light jogging, leisure biking, and hiking, rather than strenuous outdoor running sports. Swimming is often recommended for asthmatics because of its many positive factors: a warm, humid atmosphere, year-round availability, and the body's horizontal position, which may help to mobilize mucus from the bottom of the lungs. (In fact, some Olympic swimmers have severe asthma.)

   Other activities recommended include sports that involve using short bursts of energy, such as baseball, football, wrestling, short distance track and field events, golfing, gymnastics, and surfboarding. Cold weather events, such as cross-country skiing and ice hockey, or long-distance, non-stop activities like basketball, field hockey, or soccer are not recommended, as they are more likely to aggravate airways. However, many asthmatics have found that with proper training, care, and prescribed medications, they are able to excel at any sport.

*continues*

continued

2. Drugs administered prior to exercise, such as albuterol, metoproterenol, terbutaline, cromolyn sodium, nedocromil, and theophylline are all helpful treatment options in controlling and preventing exercise-induced bronchospasm. However, it is very important for everyone with exercise-induced asthma to have a breathing test at rest to assure that they do not have undiagnosed chronic asthma.

3. Athletes should restrict exercising when they have viral infections, when pollen and air pollution levels are high, or when temperatures are extremely low.

4. It is important to do warm-up exercises and stretches before exercising. These make for a safer workout, since they slowly increase breathing levels and alleviate chest tightness.

## CONCLUSION

For years, asthmatic children and adults felt that they could not take part in team and recreational sports or vigorous activities. Today, with proper detection and treatment, those affected by exercise-induced asthma and bronchospasm can participate on a level playing field with those who do not have asthma. People with asthma can become accomplished in a wide variety of sports, exercise, and recreational activities, which are beneficial to both physical and emotional health and well-being.

**NOTES:**

Courtesy of American Academy of Allergy, Asthma and Immunology, 1-800-822-2762, www.aaaai.org.

# Asma inducida por ejercicio y broncoespasmo

Hasta un 85% de asmáticos tienen síntomas de sibilancias durante o después del ejercicio. Además muchos pacientes no asmáticos con alergias o antecedentes familiares de alergia presentan broncoespasmo o sensación de opresión de las vías respiratorias causadas por el ejercicio. Otros síntomas incluyen latidos acelerados del corazón, tos, y opresión del tórax que ocurren de cinco a diez minutos después del ejercicio.

La exposición al aire frío y a la baja humedad tiende a empeorar los síntomas ya que se cree que ambos aumentan la pérdida de calor de las vías respiratorias. La obstrucción nasal empeora el asma inducida por ejercicio ya que el aire inspirado no es humedecido y calentado en la nariz. Los contaminantes ambientales (como el dióxido de sulfuro), altos niveles de polen e infecciones virales de las vías respiratorias también aumentan la gravedad de las sibilancias después del ejercicio.

### Actividades que causan sibilancias
(En orden de gravedad)

1. Carrera libre (la más probable para inducir asma);
2. Carrera en banda sin fín;
3. Ciclismo;
4. Natación (la menos probable de inducir síntomas).

### Exámenes

1. Se efectúa historia clínica del paciente;
2. Se efectúa prueba respiratoria mientras el paciente se encuentra en reposo para ver si tiene asma sin diagnosticar. Esta prueba deberá repetirse después del ejercicio;
3. Podrían efectuarse pruebas especializadas que pueden incluir ciclismo, carrera y pruebas de esfuerzo en banda sin fín.

### TRATAMIENTO

1. Selección cuidadosa del ejercicio como caminar, trote ligero, ciclismo sin esfuerzo, y caminatas largas pueden ayudar a aquellos que no pueden tolerar deportes como carreras extenuantes al aire libre.

(Sin embargo es importante recordar que la mayoría de los pacientes con asma o broncoespasmo inducido por ejercicio deberán recibir pre-tratamiento con medicamentos adecuados para permitirles participar en cualquier actividad que ellos elijan.)

*continúa*

continuación

La natación es frecuentemente considerada el deporte de elección para asmáticos y para aquellos con una tendencia hacia el broncoespasmo a causa de sus muchos factores positivos: un ambiente caluroso, húmedo, disponibilidad durante todo el año y el modo en que la posición horizontal podría ayudar a movilizar el moco de la parte inferior de los pulmones. La natación también tonifica los músculos superiores del cuerpo.

Otras actividades recomendadas para asmáticos incluyen deportes que involucran el uso de descargas cortas de energía, tales como el beisbol, futbol, luchas, carreras de campo y pista de corta distancia, golf, gimnasia y surfear en tablas.

Eventos en clima frío (tales como esquiar y hockey sobre hielo) o actividades contínuas sin descanso (como basketball, hockey de campo o soccer) son más probables que afecten las vías respiratorias. Sin embargo muchos asmáticos han encontrado que con entrenamiento adecuado y cuidados médicos, pueden sobresalir como corredores o aún como jugadores de basquetball.

2. Medicamentos administrados antes del ejercicio, tales como salbutamol, metaproterenol, terbutalina, cromoglicato, nedocromil y teofilina son opciones útiles de tratamiento para controlar y prevenir el broncoespasmo inducido por ejercicio. Sin embargo, es muy importante para todos los pacientes con asma inducida por ejercicio que se les efectúen pruebas respiratorias en reposo para descartar la posibilidad que padecen de asma crónica.

3. Los atletas deben reducir el ejercicio cuando tengan enfermedades virales, cuando los niveles de polen y contaminación estén altos o cuando la temperatura sea extremadamente baja.

4. Ejercicios de calentamiento antes de competencias son importantes y han demostrado alivio para la opresión torácica.

5. El fruncir (entrecerrar) los labios para respirar podría también ayudar a reducir la obstrucción de las vías respiratorias.

## CONCLUSIÓN

Durante años, la incapacidad para participar en programas atléticos y/o deportes de recreo ha sido un obstáculo para niños y adultos asmáticos. Se pensaba que los asmáticos no podrían y no deberían tomar parte en equipos deportivos y actividades vigorosas. Actualmente, con detección adecuada y tratamiento, aquellos afectados con asma inducida por ejercicio y broncoespasmo son capaces de hacer ejercicio el cual es benéfico para su salud física así como para su bienestar emocional.

Courtesy of American Academy of Allergy, Asthma and Immunology, 1-800-822-2762, www.aaaai.org.

## 9. Patient Pathway and Care Planning

Forms

# Patient Pathway for Pediatric Ambulatory Asthma—4/5 Years and Older

| | First Visit | Second Visit | Third Visit | Fourth Visit | Fifth Visit |
|---|---|---|---|---|---|
| Date | | | | | |
| Assessment | Your provider will physically examine you with special attention to your chest and breathing | Your provider will do a short physical examination, taking note of your lung sounds and breathing | Your provider will do a short physical examination, taking note of your lung sounds and breathing | Your provider will do a short physical examination, taking note of your lung sounds and breathing | Your provider will do a short physical examination, taking note of your lung sounds and breathing |
| Testing and Treatments | You may need a few blood tests and a chest X-ray if you do not have recent ones in your chart If you are having difficulty breathing you may get a treatment with a medication to open your airways | You will check your peak flow in the office If you are having difficulty breathing you may get a treatment with a medication to open your airways | You will check your peak flow in the office If you are having difficulty breathing you may get a treatment with a medication to open your airways | You will check your peak flow in the office If you are having difficulty breathing you may get a treatment with a medication to open your airways | You will check your peak flow in the office If you are having difficulty breathing you may get a treatment with a medication to open your airways |

*continues*

**Pediatric Ambulatory Asthma** continued

| | First Visit | Second Visit | Third Visit | Fourth Visit | Fifth Visit |
|---|---|---|---|---|---|
| Date | | | | | |
| Medications | If you have not started using an inhaled steroid (a pump) for prevention, you will begin using one at this visit<br>Inhaled steroids are like armor—they protect your lungs from injury and damage<br>You will continue using your rescue pump:<br>• Whenever you need to open airways and<br>• Before your inhaled steroid pump to open airways and help the inhaled steroid medicine work better<br>We will guide management of any prednisone taper and other asthma medications, if any | You will continue using your inhaled steroid on a daily basis<br>As you use your inhaled steroid regularly you may need to use your rescue pump less frequently<br>We will continue to adjust your other asthma medicines | You will continue using your inhaled steroid on a daily basis, adjusting the number of puffs up or down according to your peak flow diary<br>As you use your inhaled steroid regularly you may need to use your rescue pump less frequently<br>We will continue to adjust your other asthma medicines | You will continue using your inhaled steroid on a daily basis<br>You will continue to make fine adjustments in the numbers of puffs in order for you to maintain your personal best peak flow<br>As you use your inhaled steroid regularly you may need to use your rescue pump less frequently<br>We will continue to adjust your other asthma medicines<br>You will know when you need to begin oral steroids at home for any flare-ups of asthma | You will continue using your inhaled steroid on a daily basis<br>You will take the smallest number of puffs necessary to maintain your personal best<br>By now you have used your inhaled steroid regularly for several weeks—you may need few puffs of your rescue pump<br>You will use the minimal doses of asthma medicines to maintain your peak flow in the green zone and feel free of symptoms<br>You will know how to begin and taper oral prednisone when necessary to prevent your asthma from worsening |
| Consulting Physicians and Other Services | If anyone in the family smokes, he or she can be referred to a smoking cessation program | A Visiting Nurse Association nurse may visit your home to do a home assessment for asthma if some aspects of your home survey were not clear<br>Your provider will begin communication with school health services | If you seem to be bothered by allergies, you may be referred to an allergist for skin testing<br>Other types of allergy testing and evaluation for possible immunotherapy (allergy shots) may be performed | If you are interested you will be given information about local asthma support groups | |

continues

**Pediatric Ambulatory Asthma** continued

| | First Visit | Second Visit | Third Visit | Fourth Visit | Fifth Visit |
|---|---|---|---|---|---|
| Date | | | | | |
| Your Responsibilities | You will practice using your pump with or without a spacer<br><br>You will complete a home survey and bring it back completed at your next visit<br><br>You will know your best peak flow | You will practice using your pump with or without a spacer<br><br>You will receive a peak flow meter and instructions on how to use it<br><br>You will learn how to complete a home diary of your asthma and peak flow results<br><br>You will know your best peak flow | You will practice using your pump with or without a spacer<br><br>You will fill out your asthma diary twice a day; include your peak flow results, asthma problems, and any increase or decrease in doses or puffs of medicine<br><br>You will know your best peak flow | You will practice using your pump with or without a spacer<br><br>You will continue to fill out your asthma diary on a twice daily basis<br><br>You will know your best peak flow and ranges for green, yellow, and red zones | You will practice using your pump with or without a spacer<br><br>You will maintain your peak flow diary<br><br>You will know your best peak flow and ranges for green, yellow, and red zones |
| Your Understanding of Asthma and What You Will Be Learning | You will learn what happens to lungs and breathing when asthma occurs<br><br>You will learn about the several different kinds of medicines used for treatment of asthma and how they work<br><br>You will also learn how to prevent harmful side effects of these asthma medicines | You will learn how to use a peak flow meter at home<br><br>You will learn how to fill out a daily asthma diary<br><br>You will learn about the triggers of asthma and possible warning signs<br><br>You will learn how you may be able to avoid some asthma triggers | You will learn how to use your diary to prevent asthma from getting worse and to set up asthma zones: green, yellow, and red<br><br>You will learn about some improvements in your home that can decrease asthma problems<br><br>You will learn how to use your pump before playing sports and other activities | You will learn how an asthma management plan can help you make decisions to take care of asthma problems<br><br>Your asthma management plan includes when and how to use extra medications or nebulizer treatments at home, when to call your provider, and when to go immediately to the emergency department | We will review many of the topics we covered in previous visits and spend time answering your questions and concerns |

*continues*

**Pediatric Ambulatory Asthma**  continued

| | First Visit | Second Visit | Third Visit | Fourth Visit | Fifth Visit |
|---|---|---|---|---|---|
| Date | | | | | |
| Your Activity Level | At this time you (your child) may be experiencing intermittent chest tightness and shortness of breath frequently limiting activities<br><br>Asthma may cause waking during the night with shortness of breath<br><br>Asthma may cause frequent coughing | You (your child) should notice improvement in breathing and ability to play and participate in physical activities<br><br>You should notice less nighttime waking with breathing problems<br><br>You should notice only occasional coughing | You should notice more improvement in physical activity level, especially with premedicating for sports and strenuous activities<br><br>You should notice infrequent nighttime symptoms<br><br>You should notice infrequent cough | You should notice more improvement in physical activity level, especially with premedicating for sports and strenuous activities<br><br>There should be rare nighttime symptoms<br><br>There should be rare cough | You (your child) will fully participate in home, sport, and school activities with no physical limitations<br><br>There will be no nighttime symptoms<br><br>There will be no cough |
| Your Questions and Additions | Questions:<br><br>1.<br><br>2.<br><br>3. | Questions:<br><br>1.<br><br>2.<br><br>3. | Questions:<br><br>1.<br><br>2.<br><br>3. | Questions:<br><br>1.<br><br>2.<br><br>3. | Questions:<br><br>1.<br><br>2.<br><br>3. |

Source: Rufus S. Howe, *Clinical Pathways for Ambulatory Care Case Management*, Aspen Publishers, Inc., © 1996.

# Sample Care Path: Patient Version

*This form for use with adult chronic obstructive pulmonary disease/asthma contains options for patient individualization. The care path is to be used as a guideline only and does not necessarily imply a standard of care.*

*All assigned registered nurses are responsible to update, review, and sign the patient care path each shift.*

| Interdisciplinary Care Path:<br><br>**ADULT COPD/Asthma**<br><br>Expected Length of Stay: 4 days | This Plan of Care has been discussed with patient/significant other. Date: _____.<br>Signature: _____, RN<br>If discussed with someone other than the patient, specify.<br>Name: _____ Relationship _____<br>If "NA," explain: _____ | Addressograph |
|---|---|---|

| Patient Care Problems | Patient Outcomes | INTERVENTIONS | | | | |
|---|---|---|---|---|---|---|
| | | Date:<br><br>**Emergency Dept.** | Date:<br><br>**Admission Day** | Date:<br><br>**Day 2** | Date:<br><br>**Day 3** | Date:<br><br>**Day 4** |
| 1. Impaired gas exchange related to the disease process. | 1. The patient will communicate comfort in breathing.<br>\_ Date: _____<br><br>*If not achieved, write a narrative note.* | \_\_ Bedrest; positioned for optimal comfort and air exchange<br>\_\_ No caffeine<br>\_\_ Chest X-ray<br>\_\_ BUN, CBC, Lytes, Creatinine, Glucose<br>\_\_ Peak Flow, Oximetry<br>\_\_ Theophylline level<br>\_\_ ABG<br>\_\_ EKG for severe COPD<br>\_\_ IV/PO corticosteroids<br>\_\_ IV/PO aminophylline<br>\_\_ Antibiotics if suspect infection<br>\_\_ Oxygen<br>\_\_ Nebulizer/MDI<br><br>☐ No Admission | \_\_ Bedrest: positioned for optimal comfort and air exchange.<br>\_\_ No caffeine<br>\_\_ Peak Flow<br>\_\_ Oxygen<br>\_\_ Nebulizer/MDI | \_\_ BRP with assist and ad lib if tolerated.<br>Provide portable oxygen.<br>\_\_ No caffeine<br>\_\_ Oxygen<br>\_\_ Peak Flow AM<br>\_\_ Peak Flow PM<br>\_\_ Oximetry<br>\_\_ Theophylline level<br>\_\_ Convert to PO meds | \_\_ BRP ad lib if tolerated.<br>Provide portable oxygen.<br>\_\_ No caffeine<br>\_\_ Peak Flow AM<br>\_\_ Peak Flow PM<br>\_\_ Oximetry on room air if $O_2$ sat is greater than 95% on oxygen<br>\_\_ DC oxygen if indicated<br>\_\_ Convert to PO meds | \_\_ Ambulate ad lib if tolerated.<br>Provide portable oxygen.<br>\_\_ No caffeine<br>\_\_ Peak Flow AM<br>\_\_ Peak Flow PM<br>\_\_ Oximetry on room air if $O_2$ sat is greater than 95% on oxygen<br>\_\_ DC oxygen if indicated, or home on oxygen<br>\_\_ Convert to PO meds |
| 2. Knowledge deficit related to disease process and self-management. | 2. The patient/significant other will communicate understanding of disease process, treatments, and follow-up care.<br>\_ Date: _____<br><br>*If not achieved, write a narrative note.* | \_\_ Implement Emergency Department Teaching Guideline | \_\_ Patient/family assessment<br>\_\_ Implement Learning Checklist for Compromised Respiratory Status | \_\_ Patient/family assessment<br>\_\_ Implement Learning Checklist for Compromised Respiratory Status<br>\_\_ Patient/family assessment<br>\_\_ Continue Learning Checklist for Compromised Respiratory Status<br>\_\_ Evaluate for MDI conversion & teaching: B-agonist, inhaled steroids<br>\_\_ Evaluate for DME, HH, SNF<br>\_\_ Discuss discharge date with physician | \_\_ Patient/family assessment<br>\_\_ Continue Learning Checklist for Compromised Respiratory Status<br>\_\_ Evaluate for MDI conversion & teaching: B-agonist inhaled steroids<br>\_\_ Evaluate for DME, HH, SNF<br>\_\_ Discuss discharge date with physician | \_\_ Finalize arrangements<br>\_\_ Complete Learning Checklist for Compromised Respiratory Status in preparation for discharge tomorrow |
| | | GRASP: 8am-4pm \_\_\_\_ | GRASP: 8am-4pm \_\_\_\_ | GRASP: 8am-4pm \_\_\_\_ | GRASP: 8am-4pm \_\_\_\_ | GRASP: 8am-4pm \_\_\_\_ |

*continues*

**Sample Care Path: Patient Version** continued

| Emergency Dept. | | | Admission Day | | | Day 2 | | | Day 3 | | | Day 4 | | |
|------|------------|-------|------|------------|-------|------|------------|-------|------|------------|-------|------|------------|-------|
| INIT | PRINT NAME | TITLE | INIT | PRINT NAME | TITLE | INIT | PRINT NAME | TITLE | INIT | PRINT NAME | TITLE | INIT | PRINT NAME | TITLE |
|  |  |  |  |  |  |  |  |  |  |  |  |  |  |  |
|  |  |  |  |  |  |  |  |  |  |  |  |  |  |  |
|  |  |  |  |  |  |  |  |  |  |  |  |  |  |  |
|  |  |  |  |  |  |  |  |  |  |  |  |  |  |  |

| INSTRUCTIONS FOR USE: *Initial* if intervention *initiated* *Leave blank* if intervention *not initiated* *Write NA* if intervention *not applicable* | If the intervention is not initiated within 24 hours, document a narrative note. A narrative note is not required for "NA" (not applicable). | DAY SHIFT assures that the Care Path is reviewed and variances are documented. | Discharge to: Home ☐  SNF ☐  HH ☐  SOC ☐ Date: _____ Time: _____ SOC: _____ |
|---|---|---|---|

Source: Donna Cramer and Susan M. Tucker, "The Consumer's Role in Quality: Partnering for Quality Outcomes," *Journal of Nursing Care Quality*, Vol. 9:2, Aspen Publishers, Inc., © January 1995.

# Sample Patient Standard of Care Information Sheet

**INFORMATION ABOUT YOUR PLAN OF CARE**
**Compromised Respiratory Status (BREATHING PROBLEMS)**

> 1. **We will make a plan of care to meet your basic care needs.**
> 2. **It is important that you and your family let us know about any questions or concerns.**
> 3. **We will provide a safe and clean environment.**
> 4. **We will help you understand your condition and treatments.**
> 5. **You will be asked to participate in your care.**
> 6. **We will help you plan for your continued care.**

Addressograph

| Patient Care Issues | What We Will Do | What You Can Do | Expectations |
|---|---|---|---|
| You need information about your condition. | Health care team members will provide you with information about your condition.<br><br>We will tell you about treatments, medicines you receive, and follow-up care. | Please ask any questions about your treatment and follow-up care. Let us know if you do not understand something we say. | You will have information you need and want about your treatment plan. |
| What will happen to you during your hospitalization. | We will take your temperature, pulse, and blood pressure as needed. We may need to wake you at night.<br><br>We may weigh you every day and keep track of how much you eat and drink and how much you urinate.<br><br>You may be on a special diet.<br><br>We will give you medications as your physician orders. Most medicines are given by mouth or through a needle in one of your veins. | Help us keep track of what you eat, drink, and urinate.<br><br>Ask us any questions you have about your diet.<br><br>If you have a needle in your vein, tell the nurse right away if you feel any burning or discomfort when medicine is going through the needle or if you see any swelling around the needle. | You will understand the treatments and activities you experience in the hospital. |
| You may have shortness of breath or feel extremely tired. | The physician may ask us to give you respiratory treatments, oxygen, and medicines to help your body get rid of extra fluid. | Let us know if your shortness of breath gets worse or you have chest pain. | Our goal is for you to become less short of breath and be able to resume your normal activity gradually without feeling tired. |

*continues*

**Sample Patient Standard of Care Information Sheet** continued

| Patient Care Issues | What We Will Do | What You Can Do | Expectations |
|---|---|---|---|
| You may experience discomfort. | We will ask you if you are having discomfort.<br><br>We will give you medication for your discomfort as you request and as your physician has ordered. | If you start to have discomfort, tell the nurse before it becomes too severe.<br><br>If you feel no relief 30 minutes after you have received medication, tell the nurse. | Your discomfort will be controlled or relieved at a level acceptable to you. |
| Planning for your continued care. | We will ask you about any special needs you have at home.<br><br>We will give you written instructions about medications, diet, activity, and things you need to report to your physician.<br><br>We will assist you to schedule your follow-up visits with your physician. | Tell us about any concerns or needs you have.<br><br>Review the instructions we give you; ask about anything that is unclear before you leave. Follow instructions about diet closely.<br>Take your medicines as directed.<br>Avoid smoking, alcohol intake, and stressful situations. | You will be able to care for yourself at home and gradually increase your activity.<br><br>You will know who to call for questions and concerns. |

## NOTES:

Source: Donna Cramer and Susan M. Tucker, "The Consumer's Role in Quality: Partnering for Quality Outcomes," *Journal of Nursing Care Quality,* Vol. 9:2, Aspen Publishers, Inc., © January 1995.

# Index